✳

Aromatherapy and Your Emotions

Aromatherapy and Your Emotions

SHIRLEY PRICE

Thorsons

Thorsons
An Imprint of HarperCollins*Publishers*
77–85 Fulham Palace Road
Hammersmith, London W6 8JB

The Thorsons website address is www.thorsons.com

Published by Thorsons 2000

10 9 8 7 6 5 4 3 2 1

A catalogue record for this book is available
from the British Library

ISBN 0 7225 3862 6

Printed by Caledonian International
Book Manufacturing Ltd, Glasgow

Contents

Acknowledgements

To my husband Len, for his devoted help, love and encouragement throughout. Thanks also to Robert Stephen who read through the finished manuscript and gave helpful suggestions. As I don't know Anne Infante personally, I would like to thank my friend George Cranley for introducing me to her cassette.

Lastly, but by no means least, my thanks go to God, without whose presence and guiding help it would have been impossible to finish the book in the allotted time – or to arrive at the down-to-earth reasoning for the choice of essential oils which could help the emotions.

Author's Note

Since the age of 30 I have adopted a positive attitude to life in general and to my health in particular. In writing this book my aim and belief is that it will help others to achieve better health by encouraging in them a similar positive attitude, assisted by the appropriate use of those wonderful natural agents, essential oils.

To this end my pen has targeted the bright, the cheerful and the optimistic in preference to the dull, the dismal and the pessimistic. I feel, therefore, at one with the sentiment expressed by Jane Austen in her novel *Mansfield Park*, where we find the words

'Let other pens dwell on guilt and misery'

1 *Emotions – What They Are and How They Affect Us*

When dealing with people remember you are not dealing with creatures of logic, but with creatures of emotion, creatures bristling with prejudice, and motivated by pride and vanity.

Dale Carnegie

By starving emotions we become humourless, rigid and stereotyped; encouraged, they perfume life; discouraged, they poison it.

Joseph Collins

What Are Emotions?

The concept of emotions is difficult to pin down. I know you will understand that my interpretation of (and views on) something as intangible and delicate as emotions may not be the same as someone else's, and this needs to be borne in mind whilst reading this book. Each of us is an individual – and nowhere is this more evident than when looking into the fascinating area of the mind. In aromatherapy, the health of the mind is given equal importance to the health of the body:

Aromatherapy is the controlled and informed use of plant essential oils to protect and improve the general health and well-being of the whole person – body, mind and spirit.

It is relatively easy to explain, and see, bodily health, but not so easy to explain or see mental health, yet they are very closely linked. I hope to show just how much the mind and the spirit, through the emotions, are able to affect the physical body towards good or ill health – and how emotions which prove to be detrimental to one's health can be eased and comforted by using essential oils. It would be beneficial to begin by trying to understand the meanings of mind and spirit – and, of course, emotion.

My definition of aromatherapy, given above, is particularly important here. Too many people believe it only to be 'a massage using essential oils'. This definition is narrow, restrictive and incomplete; if it were truly the definition, it would be much more difficult for people at home to make full use of these wonderful volatile extracts from plants, precluding as it does the many simple and effective ways (which are fully explained in Chapter 9) available to them for using essential oils in the home.

The Mind

In all my other books, I have concentrated principally on the effect of essential oils on the *physical* body, with only a small part being devoted to their effects on the mind – let alone the spirit! However, the beneficial effect that essential oils can have on the mind lends an added dimension to their use in healing (Price, 1991), so let's take a look first at the definition of the mind. In my pocket dictionary it appears as:

> that which thinks, perceives, feels, etc.; the seat of consciousness; the site of memory or remembrance; where opinion is formed before its verbal expression; reason, sanity; way of thinking and feeling.
>
> Collins, 1981

The Spirit

In giving you the following definition of the spirit, I have deliberately missed out the fact that it can mean the soul (this can cause controversy between some practitioners of complementary medicines – including aromatherapy – and some narrow-minded people in the Church). I have also omitted its interpretation as a ghost or supernatural being; and my reasons for not including its meaning as a liquor go without saying! I am giving the definition of the spirit in all the remaining meanings, as these are relevant to our exploration of aromatherapy and the mind – and therefore the emotions. It is very interesting to see how two dictionaries have defined spirit:

> the thinking, feeling part of man; life, will, thought, etc. regarded as separate from matter; disposition, mood; vivacity, courage, etc.
>
> Collins, 1981

> The principle of thought; actuating emotion, disposition, frame of mind.
>
> Chambers, 1991

Emotion

Have you ever tried to explain the word 'emotion'? It is not easy, as I have discovered; even dictionaries give different explanations!

> strong feeling; excitement; any specific feeling, as love, hate, fear, anger, etc.
>
> Collins, 1981

> a disturbance of mind – a mental sensation or state; instinctive feelings as opposed to reason.
>
> Chambers, 1991

Both dictionaries used are right, the earlier one giving examples and the later one being more explicit.

The definition suggested by a friend of mine is that emotion is an involuntary response to a set of circumstances affecting a person; however, as people are individuals and each reacts differently, the intensity and the kind of emotion produced – and the expression of that emotion – varies greatly. The variation between people is so wide that it is not possible for an observer to judge the depth of feeling experienced by the individual (Stephen, 1999).

Another helpful definition is that emotion is both a psychic and a physical reaction (as anger or fear) subjectively experienced as strong feeling – and physiologically involving changes that prepare the body for immediate vigorous action (Merriam-Webster, 1994).

Emotions are certainly extremely personal and are not experienced in the same way by everyone; as one of the Proverbs in the Bible (14:10) says:

> Your joy is your own; your bitterness is your own. No-one can share it with you.

The Wingates (father and son) also expressed it very well in their medical encyclopaedia (1988):

> much misunderstanding comes from supposing that emotions are (or should be) the same for everyone, or that normal and abnormal physical responses to emotion can be defined.

Did you notice the following similarities in the definitions?

- 'mind' began and ended with thinking and feeling
- 'spirit' began also with thinking and feeling; and
- 'emotion' also included the word feeling.

To me this is important, because it echoes my own view that these three concepts are intertwined; it also shows that mind and spirit (especially for complementary therapy treatments) are inextricably linked – they are almost one. It is almost as though the mind is where the spirit lives; a thinking and feeling 'home', the dwelling place for consciousness, which my dictionary interprets as 'awareness; the totality of one's thoughts, feelings and impressions'. Incidentally, Robert Stephen tells me that this corresponds with the Hebrew view, where there are only two elements to the one person – the physical and the spiritual/emotional/intellectual. It becomes even more complex when you realize that in the east, the seat of the emotions (Tan Den) is situated in the centre of the abdomen, but that, in the first century, the seat of the emotions was the bowels, not the heart or the solar plexus as is the accepted view nowadays.

The home referred to above has several rooms:

- one for memory and remembrance (a sort of library), for facts and emotions previously experienced, i.e. our subconscious mind;
- one for forming an opinion, where we can sort out our thoughts before expressing them – a room where we rarely go (unfortunately) before we respond to someone with whom we are angry;
- one for finding our sanity and where we could reason with ourselves;
- one where our spirit could go when it has to decide how to deal with disposition and mood, or any other thought or feeling (emotion – remember the definition of that?) about which it is not sure;
- and one room which is secret – a room which our unconscious mind has all to itself.

To show you how essential oils can make a big impact on this home – in all its rooms – we first need to find out how they can find their way into the brain, where this 'home' is situated. The capacity of the brain is enormous; we presently use only about a tenth of the power of which it is capable, and it has been referred to as our computer (Hay 1988, p.157) or switchboard. It is up to us to direct our minds to press the keyboard of this 'computer' positively, to produce the desired words or pictures on our mental screen. Essential oils and their aromas have a very special part to play in the emotions we feel. All the senses have their impact on our emotional state, but the sense of smell is unique and different from the other senses in that it has direct connection with the emotional centre in the brain, the limbic system. Chapters 3 and 4 are devoted to these two fascinating stories – the aroma pathway to the brain and the dynamics of positive thought in the mind/body relationship.

Sweet scents are the swift vehicles of still sweeter thoughts.
Walter Savage Lander

How Emotions Affect Us

Emotions affect different people in different ways; it depends on what sort of person you are – for example, your moral beliefs, how active a conscience you have. Herbert Vander Lugt suggests that the idea that we are not accountable to anyone – not even to God –

appeals to many people. But he also believes that this contradicts the deep-down feeling (which we call our conscience) that there are some things we should do and some things we should not do (Vander Lugt, 1999). For example, a basically moral person would feel guilty if stealing something, however small, and experience fear while doing it. A basically amoral (and, of course, an immoral) person, on the other hand, would feel elation rather than fear – for having 'got away with it'. It is the same with sex nowadays. For many people, it is a 'game' – a 'must have' – and shame, fear or guilt are no longer the emotions connected with clandestine sex.

Believing and trusting in God, Divine Creator, a Higher Being or Universal Power (the latter three of which, in my opinion, are simply other names for God), also makes a difference to behaviour, and therefore to emotional experiences to some extent. Without belief in Something or Someone being responsible for the creation of the world and all that is amazing, beyond comprehension and wonderful within it – from a complex human being to a simple daisy – unhappy people could possibly experience despair. On the other hand, those who *do* have a belief of some sort would automatically have hope, and believe that things could improve for them. Such people are more likely to respect their fellow humans and less likely to suffer from emotions such as greed, lust, hate or anger to a degree that would harm another person.

In my experience, life is both richer and kinder when following a moral code. We do not have to be 'religious' to live a life which includes consideration for others, and all the major faiths (Islam, Buddhism, Judaism, Christianity, etc.) propose a way of life which is beneficial both to a person's well-being and to those around them.

I remember, as I am sure do many of us who are grandparents now, that when we were young our parents didn't have to lock any doors, or close the windows, before going out. I also remember going to the park with my elder sister – without our parents – when she was only 12, and going for walks in places where now parents could not possibly let their children go alone without pangs of anxiety and worry. Fear, in these respects, was not an emotion as frequently experienced as it is nowadays.

So there is much to consider when trying to understand the emotions – it can be quite complicated! One thing, however, is certain –

emotions influence perception, learning and memory and empathic, altruistic and creative actions (*Encyclopaedia Britannica*, 1996).

Clive Wood (1990, pp.46–49) tells us that when psychologists talk about emotion, they often refer to it as *affect*. Positive and negative affect can be measured on a scale (called the Bradburn Affect Scale after its creator) and people who have been asked questions relating to their feelings have been found to experience positive emotions most of the time:

- 'positive affect' moods can vary from feeling interested, delighted, enthusiastic and excited – down to feeling sleepy, tired and 'worn out'
- 'negative affect' moods can vary from feeling at ease and calm – down to feeling hostile, disturbed and upset.

Grouping Emotions

Emotions can be classed in several ways, though the first of the following possibilities is the one I prefer – it prevents discussion on what is and is not negative, as several so-called 'negative' emotions can, under certain circumstances, be 'positive' and vice versa.

Primary and Secondary Emotions

Primary emotions are usually considered to be grief, fear, anger, guilt and jealousy. Secondary emotions include apathy, moodiness, confusion, timidity, inferiority, etc. Primary emotions can also be welcome ones, like peace, joy and love, etc., although *because* these are pleasant, they do not generally feature in books giving advice on how to handle one's feelings. Also, even pleasant feelings, like most things, can be bad if carried to excess – love can turn into obsession; excessive joy can become destructive – the balance between good and bad emotions can be very delicate.

Pleasant and Unpleasant Emotions

We each have our own idea of which emotions are pleasant and which are unpleasant. Most of us would wish to experience happiness, cheerfulness, confidence and be generally comfortable all the time. Some people would want to include tolerance, ambition, excitement, patience, faith, love of others – many would not. So although this easy personal classification needs no explanation, it is nevertheless very individual and would not be applicable to everyone.

Stressful and Stress-free Emotions

Pleasant emotions are stress-free, as perhaps are most secondary emotions, although here it would depend on the depth and intensity of the feeling. Take shyness as an example. It doesn't seem to bother some people that they are shy; some may not even feel that they are – it may be an opinion formed by the onlooker. On the other hand, shyness can affect a person to the extent that they never accept invitations to parties or go on dates, and they make a mess of every interview for a better job. In other words, their shyness causes them stress.

Productive and Destructive Emotions

These can also be viewed as 'friendly and hostile', which I rather like – or 'positive and negative'.

Productive and destructive are the names usually used when talking about emotions in a counselling situation (Vernon, 1998). Productive emotions are those which 'produce' or generate (or are produced or generated by) positive feelings about a situation, both for ourselves as well as for others – and are friendly. Destructive emotions are those which have a negative or hostile effect, 'destroying' either ourselves (emotionally – and sometimes physically as a result) or the others involved in the emotional expression.

In choosing a suitable name to describe emotions which would be in the so-called destructive group, a slight difficulty arises. Although none would be positive (as are love, joy and happiness), not all are negative. Sorrow, fear and some forms of guilt and anger may be unwanted, unpleasant or depressing – but they can also be necessary, whilst others (such as greed, selfishness, etc.) could possibly only come under the heading of 'negative'. The interesting thing about the first classification (primary and secondary) is that it allows for the emotions within each group to be either productive or destructive, positive or negative, depending on the situation and the person.

Productive emotions are primarily constructive, and are beneficial for the well-being of the person concerned. They include feelings of love, peace, calm, joy, hope, patience, cheerfulness, enthusiasm, thankfulness, faith — I am sure you can think of more! Strangely, if one were to try and make a list of productive or positive emotions, it would be much shorter than a list of destructive or negative ones. However, according to Norman Bradburn (Bradburn Affect Scale 1969), the majority of us spend our lives experiencing mostly positive emotions, which indeed, *should* be those which affect the largest part of life experience.

When I used to write an editor's letter for *The Aromatherapist*, I liked to end with six to eight words starting with the same letter, e.g. Yours *cheerfully, calmly, caringly, confidently, courteously,* etc. It was fun (I bought a baby thesaurus for speed) — I was always amazed that with many of the letters in the alphabet, hostile words frequently far outnumbered the friendly ones.

At school, we had to learn by heart 1 Corinthians: 13. It was not from one of the new translations of the Bible, and was, in my view, a more poetic version. It is quite short — and well worth reading if you have not already done so. It is all about hope, faith and love (charity, in some biblical versions, though I prefer the word love). These are all positive emotions, which, if we 'own' in our inner being, give us guaranteed peace and contentment.

> Love is patient, love is kind.
> It does not envy, it does not boast, it is not proud.
> It is not rude, it is not self-seeking, it is not easily angered, it
>   keeps no record of wrongs.
> Love does not delight in evil but rejoices in the truth.
> It always protects, always trusts, always hopes, has faith and
>   always perseveres.
> Love never fails ...
> And now these three remain; faith, hope and love.
> But the greatest of these is love.
>
> 1 Corinthians: 13

It is only when people's basic needs of food and safety have been satisfied that other emotions begin to be experienced. Love is the next most important need, the need to love someone and the need to *be* loved. It is important for us to give love, as well as to receive it – be it from parents, a friend, a wife, a husband, a partner, children. The need to give out love and the need to receive love are immensely powerful impulses which, overall, have a great influence over our lives in general.

It is my belief that if true love is part of one's being, destructive emotions like hate, arrogance, negative anger and jealousy – and therefore probably guilt – will rarely be experienced. If they are, with love, they will be easier to cope with in ourselves and easier to understand in other people.

> Love and faithfulness keep a king safe; through love his throne is made secure.
>
> Proverbs 20:28

Even fear can be affected by love; it is forgotten completely in a situation where protection of a loved one, a child (or even an animal) is paramount. We are prepared, without having to think about it, to throw ourselves into a river, into a fight or into a road full of traffic to save someone we love dearly. John, one of Jesus's disciples, was right when he said:

> There is no fear in love ... perfect love drives out fear.
>
> 1 John 4:18

Following are some positive emotions (and/or states of mind), with their opposing feelings. Almost any essential oil (or essential oil mix) – which has an aroma you really like – will maintain positive emotions already being experienced. In my *Aromatherapy Workbook* (1993), for example, I describe how essential oils enhance a happy atmosphere at a party or at Christmas. To counter any threat to your positive, productive emotions, or to maintain those you already have – such as confidence, happiness, trust, tolerance – essential oils which have a positive effect on their opposing feelings (in bold below) can be used. These *opposing* feelings/emotions and those accompanying them are discussed in detail in Chapter 7, with the relevant essential oils to help relieve or release them:

- Happiness, joy, peace – **grief**

    Extreme grief is injurious to the lungs, but joy counteracts grief
    (Veith 1992, p.120)

- Kindness, tolerance, amenability, understanding, ability to forgive – **anger**

    Anger is injurious to the liver, but sympathy counteracts anger
    (Veith 1992, p.42)

- Confidence, bravery, courage – **fear**
- Selflessness, charity, trust, acceptance – **jealousy**
- Honesty, innocence, integrity – **guilt**
- Enthusiasm, passion, stamina, persistence – **apathy**
- Composure, enlightenment, understanding, clear thinking – **confusion**
- Bravery, courage, daring, confidence – **timidity**
- Cheerfulness, amiability, constancy – **moodiness**
- Down-to-earth, factual, tangible – **airy-fairy**

Control of the Emotions

Although we don't need any help to appreciate positive emotions like happiness and joy, we can promote, augment or prolong them by using essential oils. Destructive emotions are not augmented by essential oils – rather, they are affected in a completely opposite way by being discouraged, diminished or shortened. Essential oils can play an important part in relieving or releasing destructive emotions and positive thinking helps to prevent their reoccurrence *(see Chapter 4)*.

    Civilisation demands self control, and self control is learning not to act as emotion dictates.
    Lindenfield, 1998

Controlling emotions is not an easy matter for some people, especially motorists who direct 'road rage' at other drivers! Most of us have, at some time or another, been so annoyed by something that we would have liked to 'punch' the person responsible for the particular word or action. The emotion of anger is aroused, though we would normally control ourselves sufficiently either to get back at them with words, or to control the feeling altogether – to save a serious argument. Unfortunately, when an emotion is completely repressed, it is much more likely to affect the health adversely than if cross words had been spoken. Even better for the health would be to express the emotion physically and 'get it completely out of the system', as we say! Anger is a spirited emotion, and if channelled, such as by beating the head on a cushion, the energy is released; if suppressed, it can turn inwards and become depression.

> Anger is momentary madness, so control your passion or it will control you.
>
> Horace

> The greatest remedy for anger is delay
>
> Seneca

because

> An angry man opens his mouth and shuts his eyes.
>
> Cato

As the quotations above suggest, we cannot, in this world, always act as our emotions demand and must look to ways of controlling them without repressing them – in other words, giving them relief by other means. If, however, instead of being set on a healing road, emotions are harboured or suppressed for any length of time without help, they can eventually have a detrimental effect on the health; mental attitudes play a far greater part in day-to-day health than is realized *(see 'psychoneuroimmunology' in Chapter 4)*.

Destructive Emotions

Destructive emotions are primarily harmful, being detrimental to ourselves, although not necessarily negative. When they *are* negative, their expression is detrimental to the well-being of the person to whom they are addressed.

'Destructive' may not appear at first to be quite the right word to describe the feelings and emotions we would rather not have, but when we realize that there are these two possible interpretations of the word as far as our emotions are concerned, it is easier to appreciate *(see 'Self-love' below, which also has two possible interpretations)*.

For example, if a list was made of destructive and negative emotions, there would be a greater number of destructive feelings represented than productive ones, even though destructive ones usually – and fortunately – affect us for very much shorter periods of time. However, if negative emotions begin to play too large a part in our life, we need to do something about it – and if we cannot do it alone, we will need help, either from a complementary practitioner specializing in self-help or from a book. Self-help, including cultivating positive thoughts, becomes much easier with the aid of essential oils, as the aromas alone can be beneficial to the state of mind even before self-help and positive thinking enter the scene. To put it more precisely:

- destructive emotions can damage our relationships with other people; hate, anger, selfishness and irritability, for example, adversely affect the person to whom they are directed, 'destroying' to some extent (depending on the length of time it is experienced) the regard or respect that person may have for us
- destructive emotions can also be self-destructive, affecting our own feelings and leading to a lowered immune system and ill-health if suffered or suppressed for too long.

For example:

> From the body of one guilty deed
> A thousand ghostly fears and haunting thoughts proceed.
> William Wordsworth

> Every guilty person is his own hangman.
> Seneca

> Grief is the agony of an instant: the indulgence of grief the
> blunder of a life.
>
> Benjamin Disraeli

Destructive emotions are not straightforward, some being more complicated than others. Undue stress, which is really a state of mind affecting emotions and is a recognized illness of modern life, can produce emotions which are both productive and destructive *(see Chapter 6)*.

Many emotional responses can be more or less controlled by the individual. Grief, however, is a complex emotional experience thrust upon someone without their having control over the event, and more than one emotion is involved; it has five stages – disbelief, shock, denial, anger and acceptance (Stephen, 1998).

I once read about an aromatherapist who undertook a training course in Emotional Therapy. She said that it enabled her to realize that emotions are definitely separate from the mind – and, once they start to surface, are not as easy to control as we would like to believe (Rochfort, 1998).

With positive application and belief in oneself, however, the mind can at least be persuaded to have an effect on behaviour, emotions and, therefore, health. Attitude of mind is so important that it is discussed in detail in Chapter 4. Suffice it here to say that destructive emotions, as well as being harmful and detrimental to one's well-being, can undoubtedly lead to both mental and physical ill-health. Add essential oil use to positivity and we have a sure recipe for success and good health, both mental and physical.

> People's beliefs that odours can influence their mood or health
> may lead them to perceive such consequences when they are
> exposed to an odorant – and may help trigger actual effects.
>
> Knasko, 1997

It has been said that a destructive emotion can occasionally be productive in that it can be the means to achieve a goal. For example, jealousy or envy of someone else's business success (or greed) can drive a person to achieve a successful – in the money sense – business, thus attaining their goal. Usually, however, people who have been driven by these emotions to achieve something are not usually well-liked by the community. Those who become successful without the drive of a destructive emotion are, on the other hand, usually well-liked, without even trying!

> Henry Ford said ... Thinking men know that work is the salvation of the race, morally, physically and socially; it does more than get us a living — it gets us life. However, we should not forget Jacob Marley in 'Christmas Carol', who said 'Business! Mankind should have been my business. The common welfare, ... charity, mercy, forbearance and benevolence should have been my business.'
>
> Grounds, 1999

Although we may not wish to regard destructive emotions such as greed, lust and envy as being negative, they have, since Ancient times, been among the characteristics considered best avoided, positive ones being those to aim for:

> People ... will be boastful, proud, abusive, disobedient to their parents, ungrateful, unholy, without love, unforgiving, slanderous, ... brutal, ... treacherous, rash, conceited; ... have nothing to do with them (2 Timothy 3:2–5). Strive for righteousness, ... faith, love, endurance, gentleness (1 Timothy 6:11). Do your best to add goodness to your faith; to your goodness add knowledge, to your knowledge add self-control; to your self-control add brotherly affection; and to your brotherly affection add love. These are the qualities you need (2 Peter 1:5–7).

The following two destructive emotions, hate and arrogance, have not been put into a class, nor is there a specific list of essential oils in Chapter 7 to combat them — possibly because I have never had to deal with them either in myself (as far as I know!) or in other people.

- Hate (true hate, not the hate in the frequently expressed 'I hate you!') is a complicated emotion, as it could be intertwined with jealousy, fear or even grief (having been hurt). Even anger could perhaps be involved, as both hate and anger are harsh feelings (opposites of hate are love, compassion and sympathy). To help diffuse real hate, the essential oils in the relevant categories in Chapter 7 should be tried.

- Arrogance, into whose category comes conceit, condescension and snobbery, is always negative. Pride can also be negative, when it is accompanied by haughtiness, disdain and vanity. They are all opposites of meekness, modesty, deference and humility. The essential oils to try, if it was possible to admit to these emotions, would be those which are detoxifying and cleansing, together with those which are also healing (cicatrizant) *(see Chapter 7)*.

One positive emotion I have not included is the positive form of pride, which has as its partners self-respect, dignity, self-esteem, honour, its opposites being lack of self-confidence and self-love. Essential oils to restore confidence would include relevant oils in the fear category *(see Chapter 7)* but what is vital also is a change in attitude towards yourself – and positive thinking is the concept you need *(detailed in Chapter 4)*.

Understanding Emotions

Most of us already try to live our lives conscientiously, with regard for other people. We try to 'do-as-we-would-be-done-by' and we may prefer to see the so-called destructive emotions divided into two categories:

- emotions we experience which affect only ourselves
- emotions we experience which affect others also.

This is a more personal approach and different for each of us. However, to give as clear a picture as possible on which emotions you need help with, you could make your own lists in this personal type of classification. You could then decide which of these you don't like experiencing and would like to be able to control or change. This is not an easy task, as I discovered myself long before I knew about aromatherapy.

CASE STORY

My husband and I had just started our own business and it was a struggle – a real struggle – to make ends meet. The stress (though I did not at the time know the existence of this now accepted condition) was such that I realized one day that I was always impatient or shouting at the children – or at Len. I used positive thinking to help me to be more aware of imminent incidents and try to change myself (for their sakes!). It took many months of practice and applied thinking to improve even a little bit! My reward did not come until about three years later, when my son said, after doing something for which he expected me to be angry, 'Aren't you going to say anything then? You used to be mad at me for that!'. I have continued to try to change and have found that by controlling – or changing – my destructive emotions to constructive or productive ones, my own life is calmer and happier and I have managed to banish (almost!) the guilty feelings I suffered after venting my emotions unreasonably on the other members of the family.

> A patient man has great understanding, but a quick-tempered man displays folly.
>
> Proverbs 14:29

> A soft answer turns away wrath.
>
> Proverbs 15:1

There are occasions in life when a specific action produces opposite emotions – in the doer and the receiver. Take stealing, for example. This causes destructive emotions such as sorrow, anger, frustration and often despair in innocent people, whilst the thieves (whose motive is usually greed), experience only productive emotions like satisfaction, elation and happiness, through their ill-gotten gains. They rarely experience fear; it is more like excitement – a thrilling kind of fear, which is a productive emotion. Let me tell you of an experience which illustrates how emotions differ depending on the situation and the character of the people concerned.

CASE STORY

Our neighbours in France had just been burgled when we arrived at our own house there one year. They were devastated – as anyone would be in the same circumstances. They had saved hard for their little house, which Jacques had converted from a very small barn; Jeannine made jam and wine; they had invested only a year before in a small electric generator so that they could have electric lights and a fridge – and everything, including most of their furniture, had been taken. Jacques had previously made wrought-iron grilles for his two windows and put special locks on the front door. Imagine their emotions when they arrived to find that the door had been chiselled off by the hinges! To add to their misery, they were not insured.

The emotions initially suffered by Jacques and Jeannine were all destructive – shock, despair, depression, sorrow, etc., whereas those experienced by the thieves were no doubt excitement, elation, joy (of a kind), accompanied by a feeling of triumph. It was Jacques and Jeannine who needed positive help – and essential oils – to relieve their destructive emotions and regain their normal emotional equilibrium. The thieves needed nothing – they had a positive 'reward' for their negative actions.

> The greatest incitement to guilt is the hope of sinning with impunity.
>
> Cicero

Understanding Others

Before we can begin to get to grips with human relations – knowing and understanding others – we first have to become better acquainted with ourselves. To live our lives with any degree of happiness or contentment, we must all learn to accept the destructive things about ourselves as well as the productive ones. By learning to accept ourselves we will find we can accept others.

If we see ourselves as people who reflect the value of love, this will influence our love beliefs, attitudes and behaviour towards others. If, however, our values are such that we see people only as a means towards our own ends, all the words in the world won't help us to understand them – or help them to understand us.

As each of us grew up, we acquired a set of values initially from our parents, who were the first to establish our standards of behaviour. Unfortunately, parents often expect more from a child than is reasonable. We were no doubt told that to express or even to feel anger was wrong; that we should never allow evil thoughts to enter our head; that we should always be good, not selfish or insisting on having our own way or being inconsiderate of others, but to give way to others and to the rules of society.

Most of us fall short of the ideal image our parents create for us, and this is often where guilt feelings may start creeping in. If we realize we aren't the person we thought others expected us to be, a form of self-condemnation can begin, albeit subtly, to influence our behaviour in a self-defeating way. That is why the conflict between what we are and what we feel we should be has to be resolved – or at least understood – if we are to be free enough to grow in our understanding of other people.

How many times have you read stories in the newspaper about the famous author, the brilliant actress, the empire-building businessman – all at what seems to be the very pinnacle of success – suddenly blasting their lives away with the shot of a gun, the hissing jet of a gas oven or a leap from the 39th floor? And people ask 'why?'. An amazing number of times, as the story unfolds from friends and relatives, it turns out that these people did not consider themselves successful; they had created for themselves such a lofty 'I should be' image, that they just could not possibly attain it. Examples we all know are Tony Hancock, Marilyn Monroe and Elvis Presley.

It is important to realize that what a person does, does not necessarily reflect the true person within, which is hidden from the outside world; these unhappy people had failed to reconcile their inner conflict between what they *felt* they were, what they *actually* were, and what they *aspired* to be.

Experience of life, coupled with understanding parents, teachers and friends, helps us to realize that compromise is essential to living a normal life; that it is unrealistic and beyond our reach to try to be perfect in every way, even though this may be a desirable goal. We must come to terms with our shortcomings and faults, our strengths and virtues and reach an acceptance of what we are, what we hope to be and what we can realistically achieve (which is often much more than the majority of us believe), while always striving for our ultimate goal.

Lack of Self-love, Self-confidence, Self-esteem

Many people cannot accept how they are and may regard themselves as inferior or worthless; such people do not like themselves and consequently, perhaps, are not liked by other people. People suffering from anorexia cannot accept how they are; they see themselves as fat (when in reality they are thin) and suffer because of it. Extreme emotions such as self-condemnation and inferiority complexes are destructive; the former may even cause someone to have suicidal tendencies. A surprising number of people suffer from an inferiority complex, feeling that they are not as clever or that they are less talented than their companions. This leads them to be extremely self-critical, and in an attempt to compensate, they are often too critical of other people.

A positive view of the situation could give them an emotional drive to improve themselves – and their life – with beneficial results not only for the person, but for the family and the community at large.

Loving Ourselves

The paramount emotion of love is truest when being able to love others for what they are, and not for the outward display or for what they do.

> The expression of love is perhaps one of the most important lessons that humans incarnated upon the physical plane have to learn. Without love, existence can be dry and meaningless. It is necessary that we learn to love not only those around us but also ourselves.
>
> Gerber, 1988

The Bible tells us to love our neighbours as we love ourselves. Yet it is generally felt that the emotion of loving ourselves is wrong, and that we should only cherish others in this way. To love oneself in a selfish, proud or haughty way *would* be wrong I agree; to do that would be unwise and against the general good. However, it is essential to love one's self in the *right* way and understand one's *own* emotions before one can project kind and loving emotions onto other people and understand the emotions *they* may be feeling. Only by doing this can we be useful to other people.

For example, in a life and death situation, such as in the event of an aircraft emergency, mothers are advised to put on the oxygen mask before seeing to their baby – a seemingly selfish action; however, if this is not done, both might lose their lives. Similarly, my husband, who cannot swim, would be inconsiderate of others if he jumped into a river to save someone without first putting on a life jacket, otherwise they would both perish and he would not have helped the person in difficulties (or himself!).

CASE STORY

A few years ago there were some terrible storms on the north-west coast of England. A lady was taking her dog for his usual walk along the front, when a huge wave swept the dog into the raging sea. A young policewoman, seeing the lady's distress, dived into the water to save the dog – and was drowned.

Healthy individuals are able to accept themselves as they are, without negative emotions of envy, hate, revenge or jealousy etc. playing a big part in their lives; they do not spend a lot of time wishing they were other than what they are. This is not to say that they are self-satisfied, but rather that they can accept whatever faults, flaws and deficiencies they may be aware of in themselves and can adopt a positive attitude towards improvement, taking positive action to better themselves.

It is unhealthy and unrealistic to suffer the emotions of guilt, shame, sadness or envy for something which is beyond our control, such as the way we are made, and without these unnecessary feelings we are free to move forward to a better self – and to an enjoyable life in contact with other people. Accepting our emotions enables us not only to 'see ourselves as others see us' but also to empathize and communicate with others. Once we are not fixed on our own emotions we are then able to give more support and attention to others.

Loving Yourself

Self-love does not mean 'I am better than anyone else', nor does it mean that we are more important than other people: it simply means accepting ourselves as we are, acknowledging any faults we may have – and, most important, being able to change anything we don't like, or don't want about ourselves, or which is destroying our confidence, into something we *do* like – and at each 'change', *loving ourselves a little more.*

This process also includes forgiveness – including forgiving ourselves.

> Forgiveness means accepting the core of every human being as the same as yourself and giving them the gift of not judging them ... Forgiveness starts with ourselves and extends to others.
>
> Borysenko, 1988 p.176

> Do not say 'I'll pay you back for this wrong'.
>
> Proverbs 20:22

The act of forgiving is not always easy, but is it worth ruining the rest of your life for something which a) is in the past and b) is only affecting *you* personally and not the person responsible? Forgiving them frees you from any resentment you may be nurturing, which is not doing your body or your mind any favours. *You* will be the beneficiary; you will be free – free to start living positively, free to begin loving yourself – and therefore others, starting with the person whose original action made you bitter. The more you send out loving, positive feelings to others, the more you will receive back – you will be surprised at how much – and your love of *yourself* will grow accordingly. You can now stop feeling guilty, you can stop criticizing yourself, you can forgive yourself – and life will begin to work in your favour.

The *Course in Miracles* says that 'all disease comes from a state of unforgiveness' and that 'we need to look around to see who it is that we need to forgive' (Hay 1988, p.14).

We can decide to be loving, to be forgiving and to practise 'lovingness'; however, the process starts with self-love.

Conclusion

Maybe now we can understand that we should try to discourage emotions such as

> hatred, discord, jealousy, fits of rage, selfish ambition ... and envy, and encourage in ourselves love, joy, peace, patience, kindness, goodness, faithfulness, gentleness and self control. Against such things there is no law.
>
> Galatians 5:23

With these qualities, the destructive emotions in the first part of the quote above, which are negative, are less likely to form a part of our personality or character, and the emotions which are self-destructive but not negative, such as fear, guilt, sorrow, etc., will be much easier to deal with – with the aid of essential oils. Our aim in life should be to be happy and healthy – and this is possible with love, positive thinking *(see Chapter 4)* – and essential oils!

2 What Influences
Our Emotions?

There is no doubt that events and experiences around us can influence the emotions we express or feel. Equally, the converse is true: the emotions we habitually express or feel can influence the events and experiences occurring in our lives. Let's look first at those things which can influence our emotions.

Experiences which Affect the Emotions

The emotions we feel or express can be influenced by many situations, even by the weather! Sunshine automatically lifts our spirits, making us feel happier, whilst dull, rainy weather has an opposite, depressing effect. Our lifestyle and personality (closely linked with behaviour) can also have a great influence on the emotions most often experienced. More importantly, our mind (the way we think), our health, our past experiences, touch – even aromas – all play a day-to-day role in 'deciding' which emotions are activated. Sometimes these influences are separate, but more often than not they are intertwined, more than one being involved and usually more than one emotion being experienced as a result. Let's now look at these influences in greater detail.

Lifestyle
The way we live our lives, that is to say, our lifestyle, plays a very important part in our personal development, both of the mind (including the emotions) and the body. All the following are part of lifestyle:

- the way we think and behave
- the amount of exercise we take, whether it be a sporting activity or

an individual pursuit like walking or daily workout exercises

- how many hours of sleep we allow ourselves; people's sleep needs vary, but each of us knows how much ensures that we awake refreshed and able to cope with the day ahead without becoming tired
- passive recreational pursuits; the music we listen to, the books we read, how much television we watch, the hobbies we may have (ranging from martial arts to needlework)
- the type of foods we eat; if people are in a nutritionally deprived state, their emotional well-being is likely to be adversely affected (Wallace, 1999). Chronic illnesses like arthritis and bronchitis are exacerbated by the wrong food intake and will improve with correction to the diet
- the kind of job we have; if we do not like, or are not happy in, our job, we will have a different attitude to life from those who love their work
- whether or not we have children; the responsibility of bringing up a family, whether we exert necessary discipline or don't care how they behave.

All these things affect the way we think and the emotions we experience. No complementary therapist worth his or her salt will propose a treatment without first finding out everything about the person, as, for someone to return to perfect health of both mind and body, it may be necessary to change some lifestyle 'habits'. Unfortunately, it isn't always easy – or possible – to change one's whole lifestyle; nevertheless, it is *always* possible to improve at least one aspect of it.

Past Experiences

If a child lives with criticism,
he learns to condemn.
If a child lives with hostility,
he learns to fight.
If a child lives with ridicule,
he learns to be shy.
If a child lives with shame,
he learns to be guilty.

If a child lives with tolerance,
he learns to be patient.
If a child lives with encouragement,
he learns confidence.
If a child lives with praise,
he learns to appreciate.
If a child lives with security,
he learns to have faith.
If a child lives with approval,
he learns to like himself.
If a child lives with acceptance and friendship,
he learns to find love in the world.

Anon – cited in Bennett, 1989

I am sure no child lives with every descriptive adjective listed here, good or otherwise, but there is no doubt that we have all experienced some of them and, whether assets or drawbacks, they can shape our lives and determine to a large extent how we look at ourselves and how we treat others. These emotional, psychological and spiritual influences display themselves both *in* the body (health – good or bad) and *through* the body (behaviour, attitude, etc.).

We all love to remember pleasant past experiences; they make us feel happy and we re-experience the emotions we felt at the time, be they love, joy, calm, peace, etc. Recalling an unpleasant experience, however, is not so rewarding emotionally and can reawaken emotions such as hate, anger and jealousy.

For example, children brought up with cruel and neglectful parents will, as young adults, have a totally different attitude to life (and therefore experience different emotions) from those brought up where love has radiated throughout the house. The same thing applies to those following a career they hate, suggested or forced upon them by their parents. Both will add blame to any destructive emotions which emerge as a result. It is also possible that children may reject the approach of their parents and adopt a technique with their own children which is directly opposite to their own experience. In all these cases the past will affect how these people think – their reactions and therefore their emotions – in any given circumstance.

CASE STORY

When I was at college we had a regular, but infrequent – and always unexpected – visitor to our house. She was the daughter of parents who idolized their son, but regarded their daughter as useless. They were always criticizing her, even when, after several attempts, she qualified as a nurse (her brother had become a doctor). She loved to visit my parents, who always showed her affection. It was difficult for them to do this, because Daphne's rejection had affected her behaviour – she did everything she could to gain attention. For example, one night – it was Christmas Eve and quite late – there was a knock on the door. I went to answer it, but there was no-one there. I peered round the bay window and suddenly out jumped someone – with a loud **Boo!** I had already 'jumped out of my skin' before I discovered that it was only Daphne. It turned out that she didn't want to go home because it was late and her mother would be cross, so could she stay the night?

We dreaded her rare, but impulsive, emotional visits, yet we felt intensely sorry for her – and always tried to show we were delighted to see her. One interval between visits was well over a year; her parents said she had 'got her own place' as she was 'old enough to look after herself'. On this last visit, the change in Daphne was quite remarkable. The visit, although unannounced, was 'normal' and she apologized for her erratic behaviour over the last few years. Living on her own had made a difference, she said, such that one of the other nurses (whose father was a psychologist) had discussed her previous behaviour with her – and become her friend. Four years later she was happily married to one of the male nurses at the hospital where she worked.

Dr Perry of Baylor College of Medicine in Houston, says 'experience is the chief architect of the brain' and this is true in the world of emotions too.

> For six years, Washington University psychologist Geraldine Dawson and her colleagues have monitored the brain-wave patterns of children born to mothers who were diagnosed as suffering from depression. As infants, these children showed

reduced activity ... in the area of the brain that serves as a centre for joy and other lighthearted emotions. ... She found that mothers who were disengaged, irritable or impatient had babies with sad brains. But depressed mothers who managed to rise above their melancholy, lavishing their babies with attention and playful games, had children with brain activity of a considerably more cheerful cast.

Nash, 1997

Rise Above It

What is very important to realize and accept is that what happened in the past cannot be changed (it is over and done with) and to continue to criticize or blame those responsible only nurtures further unhappiness – and resentment – without offering a solution of any kind. The solution is to push the past away and start from **now**, because what we think now shapes our future (Hay, 1998 p.35). Perhaps the parents of the children above also had a bad life; maybe they knew no different. Perhaps the parents who pushed their son into his job thought they were doing their best for him; who knows? What is sure is that long-standing resentment and criticism can prevent us from looking to a brighter future, forgiving (even if we cannot forget) and changing what we can so that we can start enjoying life. These unproductive thoughts and emotions can also adversely affect our immune system and result in eventual ill-health. I agree wholeheartedly with Louise Hay when she says, 'How foolish for us to punish ourselves in the present moment because someone hurt us in the long ago past' (Hay, 1998 p.13). Never forget that 'today is the first day of the rest of your life'.

Health

How Health Influences Emotions

The fulfilment of a person's hope in life is dependent to a large degree on the health of that person. If one is feeling stressed or depressed to the extent that it is negatively affecting the health, the emotions experienced will reflect this in proportion, with unproductive (destructive) emotions like despair, hopelessness, envy, frustration (and possibly secondary emotions like moodiness or irrationality).

The following story illustrates the influence ill-health can have on the emotions.

CASE STORY

My lovable, gentle mother (as those of you who have read *The Aromatherapy Workbook* will know) suffered for 44 years (up to her death at the age of only 74) with a crippling form of arthritis. She was rarely free of pain, even when taking painkillers. She couldn't walk, she couldn't sleep (despite her tablets) and altogether her life was a sad one. She had lost my father at the age of 62, and when in hospital with a broken hip had been totally depressed – and even angry – because *she* had lived and another lady, in good health otherwise and with a husband, had died. The proportion of destructive emotions she presented far outweighed the number of productive or positive ones and she experienced all six of the emotions mentioned above.

When people are racked with pain, cannot walk or have any other negative health condition(s), destructive emotions are more evident in their lives than productive ones. Emotions such as jealousy and envy (of people who do not 'suffer like me'), anger ('what have I ever done to deserve this?'), frustration ('I used to do that so easily'), fear ('what is going to happen to me?') and depression. It is difficult to have hope when health seems to be progressing relentlessly downhill.

How Emotions Influence Health
This is the other side of the coin, when emotions can influence the health – for good or bad. Positive and productive emotions can keep the body in good health, and negative or destructive ones can actually cause cell damage, resulting in ill-health. They can do this in two ways – consciously or unconsciously. Most people fall into the second category, unconsciously affecting their health because of the destructive, though not necessarily negative, emotions they experience on a regular basis. Such people cannot be helped until they can recognize (or realize) that they are, in fact, habitually experiencing emotions like jealousy, guilt, resentment, disapproval, etc.

> Medicine has long recognized the physiological consequences of emotional states on health, for better or for worse. Conditions like colitis ... and hypertension are well known manifestations of negative emotional states.
>
> Bennett, 1989

All illnesses can be cured, but not all patients. The writer, Harold Nicholson, once wrote that 'one of the minor pleasures in life is to be slightly ill'. Nevertheless, there are a few people who make being ill a *major* pleasure – they enjoy being ill. Their illness is not usually too serious and could easily be alleviated by a change of thinking, or by essential oils. However, they don't *want* to get completely better because their illness is able get them attention (mainly from those nearest to them).

CASE STORY

The lady who used to clean our offices had a husband with a chronic asthmatic condition. Whenever she went out with friends, he had an attack; whenever she invited a friend round, he had an attack. She asked me if essential oils could do anything to help his condition. I suggested the same oils I had used successfully on Len (my husband), with the same methods of use. She then told me he didn't believe in complementary therapies ('they couldn't possibly work') and could I suggest a method whereby he would not know they were for his benefit. She used them in a vaporizer, telling her husband they were just to give the room a nice smell. He seemed to like the aroma and Mrs N noticed too that over the next week his breathing was much easier.

However, she made the mistake of telling him he seemed better and the next day he told her to 'take this wretched stuff away – it's making me feel ill'. I then found out that he never had an attack when she went grocery shopping or went to work – only when she was doing something personal and enjoyable, or going somewhere for pleasure. He *consciously* brought on an attack to get his wife's attention, with the overriding emotion being fear – that he would get better and have to go to work, to say nothing of having to share in household duties instead of being waited on hand and foot.

If people like this really wanted to get better (and they often make a point of *saying* they do!) they could do it – by coming to grips with the emotions governing their behaviour. However, quite often, the fear of getting better – and thus losing power over others – takes hold of them. Before true healing can begin, this fear needs to be acknowledged – and treated.

Personality and Behaviour

How Personality and Behaviour Affect Emotions

The influences coming from our thoughts show themselves in every aspect of our lives. The whole personality is involved in how we think: in our relationship with other people, occupational success, prosperity, personal self-confidence, sexual relationships, whether one believes in (and perhaps uses) violence or experiences anger, guilt, fear, etc. (Bennett, 1989). Our attitude towards these things is greatly influenced by early childhood years, thus personality and behaviour cannot be completely separated from past experiences.

We obviously cannot put people into 'boxes' regarding their personality – this is another complex and individual field. However, personality types do react in different ways in the same circumstances. For example, extroverts will not feel embarrassment or fear if called upon in a theatre to come on stage to take part in a game, whereas an introvert would be very embarrassed and frightened if picked out in this way.

CASE STORY

Len and I were having lunch in our garden in France recently. A car came past and slowed down, then stopped. We did not know the people, so I thought maybe they wanted to ask us something. However, they stayed in the car, looking at our house – and us, for several minutes – just staring! I said to Len, 'We couldn't do that, could we?' Most people are like us, I think; if they wanted to look at a house or garden they were passing in the car, they would, like us, slow down a little – and perhaps stop – if no-one was there, but if the owners were there, would not dream of stopping and staring. Just the difference in personalities!

CASE STORY

Before her arthritis became so bad, my mother was a wonderful person. My father used to call her his 'angel' and he was always looking for new therapies and ideas to get her back to her original angel state. I am sure now that her suffering was responsible for some of the destructive emotions she felt and some of the amazingly ridiculous (to us) things that she did. She was exceedingly house-proud and used to keep the house like a new pin, dusting and cleaning every day, as well as doing quite a lot of entertaining. My father was a people-loving man and the meal was always followed with a sing-song round the piano as he was a gifted pianist. All this changed drastically as arthritis took over her life.

My sister and I, in our teens, had to do all the housework, including the washing and ironing, as well as following our school – and then college – studies. She did get a cleaner once, for a little while, but when we came home from college she would ask us to 'just go over' the bathroom, or stairs, or whatever, because it was not done exactly as she liked it. Perhaps the taps were not polished, or the stair rods had been missed with the duster, etc. Her personality, with its perfectionist characteristic, influenced her emotions, which when all was not right, showed irritability and impatience.

Her one big obsession was the hall floor. We had a nice, big square hall covered in linoleum, with a small Persian carpet in the middle. After we had polished this floor, we had to put brown paper over all parts of the linoleum which were walked on, to keep it clean and save us from having to do it more than once a month. If visitors came, the paper was lifted. However, she was so paranoid about keeping the floor clean that she then put newspaper over the brown paper to protect the brown paper! So we hardly ever enjoyed the beautiful shiny floor we had created with a lot of 'elbow grease'.

I didn't learn about how certain emotions and personalities can develop certain diseases until I read, several years ago now, a book called *You Can Heal Your Life* (Hay, 1988). I was amazed to read that arthritic people are 'cursed with "perfectionism", the need to be perfect at all times' (I was already aware that arthritis can develop from a continual pattern of criticism; and had worked on that myself already!) I have always been a perfectionist – about silly little things like hanging up tea towels, etc. exactly halfway on the line, so that the corners met perfectly – even if I was in a hurry! I decided to change my habits, as although I had healed myself of arthritis *(see Chapter 4)*, which began at the same age as my mother's, I didn't want anything to bring it back. I still strive for perfection, but in a different, productive, way and with a changed mental attitude.

My mother's personality also influenced her emotions to the extent that she had a continual fear of running out of commodities she might need for her cooking – she kept a duplicate of practically every item. Later, when she was on her 22 tablets a day, she suffered with an enormous fear over whether she had enough of each kind to last until the next visit of the doctor. Such was this stress that she rang up for a new supply at far too frequent intervals, regardless of how many she already had. When she died and we were clearing the house, we found tablets in her handbag, the kitchen, the bathroom, her bedroom – in fact, we collected, in all, two carrier bags full of tablets!

It is so easy for a personality to turn inwards and influence the way we feel when there is physical suffering, as the physical pain itself brings out stressful emotions. It is a vicious circle, because these emotions, in their turn, if experienced for any length of time, can also influence the personality.

Touch
Touch is a basic human behavioural need and can play not only a significant part in the attainment of good health, but can also calm turbulent emotions. If this need for touch remains unsatisfied, according to Montagu (1986), an expert on touch, abnormal behaviour will result.

In one hospital, disturbed teenagers are taught to appreciate the significance of touching and being touched, with the result that violence in the hospital has noticeably reduced (Hooper, 1988). Where essential oils and touch have been used on people with learning difficulties they become less distressed and agitated, sleep better and even 'present' themselves for massage on a therapist's day at the centre or school where aromatherapy has been introduced.

It is our thoughts which initiate touch and the touch itself is indicative of our thoughts. Touch can also convey emotions which may be difficult to express in words. Holding someone's hand, or putting our arms around them can convey more effectively than words the emotions we want to express to someone who is grieving. We use touch, too, to show how much we love someone.

Aromas

Studies have shown that aromas can influence our behaviour (Ehrlichman & Bastone, 1992) and we are surrounded every day of our lives by aromas, many of which unfortunately are synthetic. Practically every product we buy contains an aroma of some sort, from hairsprays and cosmetics to washing-up liquid and fly spray! Among natural odours are pleasant ones like flowers, and not so pleasant ones, like perspiration.

Any one of these aromas (or smells) can influence our emotions, perhaps bringing out strong, sometimes previously experienced ones, which affect us in different ways, depending on the memory the aroma revives. They can also alter our present feelings. In an article in an aromatherapy journal on the effect of aromas on emotions and moods, the writers had found, after nine years' experience, that

- fragrance can induce mood change and although this may only be slight, it is beneficial to our well-being
- fragrance can reduce stress in a person who is already stressed, although on someone without any stress the effect is minimal (Warren & Warrenburg, 1993).

Researchers in a Polytechnic Institute in America carried out experiments to see how fragrances might alter the way people think or behave. They found that those people in the room with the aroma in it set themselves higher goals and were more willing to negotiate in a friendly manner, resolving their differences more successfully, than those in the room without any fragrance (Baron, 1990).

Remembered aromas (whether consciously or unconsciously brought to mind) can have both positive and negative effects. Emotions aroused by an aroma may be different in different people according to their past experience. For instance, a man may have very pleasant associations with the aroma of a lipstick if the previous experience was a romantic evening with a pretty girl – but an unpleasant emotion may be aroused if the previous experience of that lipstick and its aroma was on a dirty glass in a restaurant.

The following story shows how an unhappy past experience was unconsciously brought to the fore by an aroma, then brought into consciousness by the listening skills of a nurse.

CASE STORY

Hospitals, as we know, have a rather special smell. When a friend of ours took his wife into hospital to have their first baby, a strange feeling came over him – a bit panicky and nauseous. He put his emotions down to worrying about the welfare of his wife during labour. However, when he went back to visit his wife (who had had a trouble-free labour) and their new-born daughter, he had the same experience – and on the following visit too. When he mentioned this to one of the nurses, she asked him if he had ever been in hospital himself. He said 'Not that I can remember.' However, his mother, who was visiting with him that day, told him that when he was two, he had accompanied his father to the hospital where his little brother was born. The nurse, who was in the middle of a course in complementary therapies, was very interested and asked his mother a few questions. Apparently, the night before he had been taken to the hospital by his father was the first time he had ever been separated from his mother and for some reason the smell of the hospital – and visiting his mother there for another two days – had been deeply embedded in his subconscious mind.

The Mind (the Way We Think)

The first thing I learned on the mind dynamics course I attended 26 years ago was that *we are not a body with a mind – but a mind that happens to have a body* and that mind is in every cell of our body; it is a part of our being – the most important part. The more we look into it, the more we can see that in the whole of life, each human being is a product of his or her own thoughts.

The influence which our thoughts (minds) exert on the emotions is apparent in every situation, whether we are conscious of it or not. In turn, our thoughts (minds) are influenced by the continually differing circumstances occurring in our everyday lives. For example:

- the way we think and behave can affect our lifestyle
- the way we think and behave can depend on our personality – and vice versa; both affect our emotions
- health can often depend on lifestyle, the opposite also being true (e.g. if a health condition puts us into a wheelchair or a hospital), but both can be affected by the way we think – and affect our emotions
- past experiences can influence our way of thinking, health, lifestyle, etc. – and although health and lifestyle cannot change the past experiences, our way of thinking is able to influence our *perception* of past experiences; again, all of these things affect how we feel – they affect the emotions
- aromas can also be linked with past experiences, pleasant or unpleasant; equally the unwanted effects of unpleasant past experiences can, whether psychological or physical, be influenced by aromas – and both have a connection to how we think, therefore affecting our emotions.

As far as the physical body is concerned, it is generally acknowledged that we are what we eat.

> If you fill your body with the right kind of food you will increase your health and vitality, improve your sense of well-being and reduce the risk of serious illness. This simple fact is the basis of naturopathy, a partnership between the healing power of nature and the self-healing ability of the body.
>
> Hartvig & Rowley, 1996 cover

We eat in order to live, but what we put into our bodies is of great importance – food gives us our energy and vitality – it is the foundation stone of our 'being' and we need to eat the best food we can to help our body to function efficiently. We all know the consequences of eating too much, when surplus energy is turned into fat we do not need. We are aware that certain foods can make us ill, that others can give us indigestion, or in some other way harm our digestive system and therefore our body. Research has confirmed that a diet high in fresh vegetables, fruits and unrefined grains can protect the body from diseases such as diverticulitis, cancer of the colon, haemorrhoids, gallstones and heart disease (Hartvig & Rowley, 1996 p.10). We choose what we eat, therefore we are responsible for the body's response to food. By eating healthy foods and saying 'no' to things which can harm us, we increase the energy and vitality of our body.

In the same way, we can choose what we think – it is our own responsibility whether we think positive, nice thoughts or negative, harmful thoughts. What a person thinks and believes will manifest itself in his or her life. Just as it is accepted that we are what we eat, it is now also accepted that we are what we *think;* we are the product of what we eat and how we think.

> Those who are continually discontented, critical of self and others (or displaying other negative emotions) are the very ones who may attract illness and personal disasters. Conversely, how many truly happy and contented people are really ill
>
> Price, 1993

Conclusion

Looking at all the things which influence the mind – and therefore the emotions, what seems to stand out, and occurs over and over again, is attitude to life. We can go on the way we are, even if not completely happy – and many people do – *or*, we can consciously change our attitude, by changing our thinking. The way we think has, I believe, the strongest influence on our lives – and hence on our emotions *(see Chapter 4)*.

3 *Aromas, Essential Oils and Their Relationship with the Emotions*

Look in the perfumes of flowers and nature
For peace of mind and joy of life.
From the writings of Wang Wei, 8th century

How Aromatherapy Affects the Emotions

Smell is the most baffling and evocative of our senses, giving us information about things we may not be able to see or hear. It has been said that 'smells seem to be plugged into our emotions', which ties in with another perfumer, who, while smelling a lemon fragrance, said 'it's not pressed lemon – it's an emotion'.

It is a well-known and proven fact that aromas can influence the health; every aromatherapy book which has been written shows how different aromas can have positive effects on particular ailments. Most of the information concerning the effects of medicinal plants on health has been collected over thousands of years of traditional use – and even though the effects of essential oils are slightly different from those of the whole plant (on account of having been distilled), many properties are similar. Essential oils have the advantage over the whole plant (especially when dried) of having the aroma concentrated sometimes as much as 100 fold and it is the aroma which we will be discussing in this chapter.

The use of scents is not practised in modern physic but might be carried out with advantage, seeing that some smells are so depressing and others so inspiring and reviving.
William Temple, Essay on health and long life, 1690

There is no doubt that when we smell an aroma it can bring about an emotion within us. Whether the emotion we feel is pleasant or unpleasant depends on:

- the nature of the smell itself; for example, everyone finds the smell of bad eggs unpleasant, whilst almost everyone is happy smelling a rose
- our previous experience of the particular aroma; the smell of petrol, although generally felt to be unpleasant, evoked in one person a feeling of enjoyment of car travel and freedom; in another person, the scent of flowers used at his father's funeral brought on an emotion of sadness. (Classen et al 1994).

This tells us that emotions evoked by smells are special to the individual, thus it is difficult to forecast what effects a given aroma may produce in any one person. Perception is affected by the blend of previous experiences and emotions – and the reaction to the smell itself.

How does such a simple thing as a smell arouse emotions, sometimes very powerful ones? Let us consider what happens inside our head and body when we come into contact with a smell. First, we are going to follow the route taken by the volatile molecules of the essential oils when they are inhaled.

An Explanation of Inhalation

Most of the healing effect of essential oils takes place primarily through inhalation, via the mind and emotional pathways. As early as 1920, two scientists, Gatti & Cayola (1923), looked at the therapeutic effects of essential oils and noted that their sedative or stimulant action was achieved more quickly through inhalation than by ingestion. They are therefore ideal tools for tackling mental and emotional states, especially if the essential oils are carefully selected on a holistic basis (Price & Price, 1999 p.149).

The process of inhalation, like every other process in our bodies, is not a simple one – it miraculously operates, as do all our bodily functions, entirely without our help, ensuring that we 'work' efficiently.

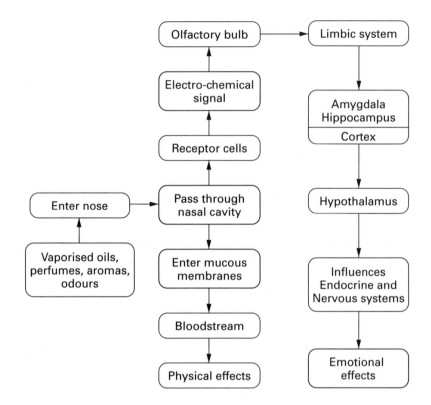

I shall give only a simple version of how inhalation works; enough for you to see how fascinating it is and also to show where emotions are found. Once essential oil molecules have found their way into the nose, two paths are followed simultaneously; some (most) of the molecules inevitably going downwards into the lungs – and some initiating signals which go upwards into the brain.

Route 1 – The Lungs
Essential oils have an immediate physical effect on the lungs and are able also to pass directly from there into the bloodstream, which carries them around the body in the blood. Because they can dissolve easily in fatty rich tissues like those of the central nervous system (CNS), the exchange of aromatic molecules from blood into such fatty tissues is facilitated (Buchbauer, 1993). Once in the blood, they

can have an effect on any organ they pass (even though they will be in a very dilute state at this time). Their action may just be revitalizing if the organ is already in good health, but if any part of the body the blood passes through is malfunctioning in any way, then the essential oils (depending on the malfunction) could have a beneficial effect.

Route 2 – The Brain

When essential oils are inhaled, aromatic molecules are also taken by the air directly to the roof of the nose, where the olfactory epithelium is situated – it is about the size of a postage stamp. In the thin layer of mucus at the top of the nose there are delicate and tiny hairlike receptors called cilia (perhaps as many as 50 million of them!) and it is here that the exchange of information begins, because each molecule has a message it wants to pass on to the brain. Each tiny cilia has countless microscopic – and different – patterns of depressions into which only a molecule of the same shape and size will fit – rather like a jigsaw – or like a key into a lock. Thus each molecule inhaled (whether an essential oil or another aroma) has to find the exact cilia which has the key to unlock its message (vanToller, 1993).

This 'lock and key' theory was first put forward by J.E. Amoore in 1962 and is the generally accepted theory of how we are able to smell, although it is not proven – and does not explain everything satisfactorily. Nor is it the only theory; Luca Turin in the BBC Horizon programme, 'Code in the Nose' (1995), suggested a different theory which says that the vibrational energy of the molecules is the critical factor in how we determine a smell. The question of just how we and other mammals are able to detect odours is believed by some to be far from settled as yet (Williams, 1996) although Dodd & Skinner (1992) are surprised to meet perfumers who believe in the vibrational hypotheses of olfactory mechanisms. We therefore do not really know exactly the mechanism by which we humans – or other animals – are able to detect smells.

We do know, however, that once a smell molecule is locked in place on the olfactory hair, its specific aromatic message is transmitted via the olfactory bulb and olfactory tract to the region of the brain linked to memory, feelings and emotions (known as the limbic system), which can trigger memory and emotional responses *(see diagram below)*. These messages are converted into action, resulting in the release of euphoric, relaxing, sedative or stimulating neurochemicals, as appropriate (Price & Price, 1999 p.150). Different aromatic molecules cause the release or blocking of specific neurotransmitters (Schmidt, 1995), which we will be mentioning later. The limbic system used to be called the rhinencephalon or 'smell brain' and it is also where past memories are stored; aromas have been used to good effect to stimulate the minds of people suffering from amnesia (Price, 1991). Suzanne Fischer-Rizzi, whom we met several years ago, writes:

> Within the limbic system resides the regulatory mechanism of our highly explosive inner life, the secret core of our being. There is the seat of our sexuality, the impulses of attraction and aversion, our motivation and our moods, our memory and creativity, as well as our autonomic nervous system.
>
> Fischer-Rizzi 1990

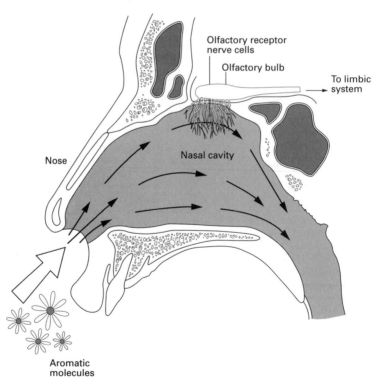

Incidentally, any molecules which are not odorous, but which are travelling up the nose, would not be able to lock on to any of the sites on the olfactory hairs, and so no sensation of smell would be created.

The number of molecules reaching the brain depends on how deeply we breathe in. With normal breathing, only a small number of molecules reach the tiny 'hairs' which transmit signals to the brain via receptor cells and the olfactory bulb *(see diagram)*. When a deep breath is taken, the impetus carries the essential oils right to the top of the nose, many more molecules are trapped by the cilia and therefore a stronger aroma is sensed in the brain.

Inhalation is by far the quickest effective route in the treatment of emotional problems because of the direct connection between the nose and the brain mentioned above. Turin (1995) says that:

> The nose is an amazing machine, which is always ready for molecules it has never seen ... That is completely different from, say, making antibodies, where you inject a molecule into somebody and a week later they are vaccinated – they make antibodies against it. With the nose there is no delay, no delay whatsoever. So it's a system that is ready for all corners, absolutely ready.
>
> Turin, 1995

The easy passage of essential oils through the blood-brain barrier is due to the fact can they can dissolve easily in fatty type substances, i.e. they are lipophilic (Buchbauer, 1993). Indeed, any substances carried by the blood to the brain have to pass through the blood-brain barrier – and it is not easily permeable. For example, medication and drugs, the majority of which are not lipophilic, have a difficult job to get through and thus produce unwanted side-effects, which is not believed to be the case with essential oils. (Essential oils do have side-effects, but these are usually favourable ones.) Because of this, the dosage of drugs or medication given by the doctor is often higher than that necessary to have a beneficial effect, and as the doctor has to be sure that his patient's condition is going to improve, he needs to prescribe a high enough dose *(see Case Story below)*. Sometimes it may be too high, but when someone's health is at stake, it is better to be sure than sorry (Rowe, 1998).

CASE STORY

When Len (my husband) was first put on his tablets for high blood pressure, he had several unwanted side-effects. Because I was lucky enough to have another doctor as a friend, we asked him if Len could perhaps try a lower dose. With the help of his wife, a nurse, who monitored his blood pressure every two or three days, he was able, by reducing the dose every three months (while using essential oils as a back up), to achieve eventually an 87.5 per cent reduction in the strength of his tablets – and all his unwanted side-effects disappeared.

He was a bit fearful (especially the night before we started), because of the uncertainty of how he would feel when we first reduced the dose – even though he was to be under daily supervision (cutting the tablet in two would give an immediate 50 per cent reduction in his medication). However, the night before, as we were preparing together those essential oils which help reduce high blood pressure (lavender, lemon, sweet marjoram and ylang ylang) for him to use with the reduced medical dose, he began to feel calmer – and because marjoram and ylang ylang also help encourage a good sleep, I gave him a tissue with these two oils to take up to bed. Not only did he sleep well, but in the morning was not at all apprehensive about our 'venture'. The following explains why:

- marjoram is calming to the nervous system and aids sleep; it seems to relax tightness in the chest – often a symptom of fear. As a respiratory tonic, it can help slow down rapid breathing, evident in the early stages. It calms and regulates the heart beat and is also a tonic to the nerves
- ylang ylang is calming and sedating and can slow down a rapid heart beat. It seems to relax fear spasms connected with the digestive system, which is adversely affected during fear.

(See Chapter 7 for full properties of both oils in all respects of fear.)

We saw in Chapter 2 how various things in our lives (health, personality, lifestyle, past experiences and aromas) can affect how we think and feel – in other words, our emotions. Aromas play a bigger part than it may appear at first glance! Of our five senses – taste, hearing, sight, touch and smell – smell has always been the one we know least about. My anatomy course at college included the anatomy of the tongue, ear, eye and nervous system – but no-one ever mentioned the anatomy of the nose and how we are able to smell, yet it is one of the most important senses we have. Even Aristotle praised the aesthetic aspect of the sense of smell, noting that pleasant odours contributed to the well-being of mankind (Ohloff, 1994 p.IX).

Smell is certainly the most subtle of our senses. It is an easy matter to cover one's ears to cut out an unpleasant noise; eyes can also be covered against something we don't want to see; we don't normally have to touch (or eat) anything we don't want to; but it is extremely difficult not to inhale a smell – after all, we have to breathe! – and normal breathing is usually through the nose. Even if we try to breathe through the mouth, some of the smell will get through. Smells refuse to be confined to any one space; they naturally spread out and diffuse into surrounding areas, mixing with other odours very easily, thus creating new aromas. Once in the brain, they act immediately on the nerve centre at the top of the nose (the cilia) and bring about an emotional reaction which may be either pleasant or unpleasant (Genders, 1972).

CASE STORY

I remember at boarding school when I discovered what the awful smell just beside the hatch into the kitchen was, because it arrived later on my plate as cabbage. Although I had previously loved cabbage when my mother cooked it at home, I didn't ever want to face cabbage again, but at this school you had to eat everything – and were made to stand on a stool all afternoon until you did eat it! After suffering this twice, I decided that as I was going to be made to eat it anyway, I might just as well have it hot. So I used to eat it while holding my nose, which took away most of the taste.

It is difficult to say which sense one would miss the most. I have always thought that the two most valued senses – and usually the most common to be lost – are sight and hearing. I must admit that had I the choice, I would find it very difficult to decide which I would prefer to keep if I had to lose one of those. Having read about a man who had lost his sense of smell I realize that whatever sense is lost would be a major misfortune. Sacks said:

> it was like being struck blind. Life lost a good deal of its savour – one doesn't realize how much 'savour' is smell. You 'smell' people, you 'smell' books, you 'smell' the city, you 'smell' the spring – maybe not consciously, but as a rich unconscious background to everything else. My whole world was suddenly radically poorer.
>
> Sacks, 1987

Is everyone's interpretation of a certain smell the same?

The answer to that question is 'No'! As I said before, every aroma is made up of many different molecules and each molecule has to have a 'slot' in which to fit. If one or two of the slots are missing, the aroma of the substance perceived is bound to be different, therefore our interpretation of an aroma is individual, and occasionally different from someone else's. Differences in sight are well recognized and are plainly visible in the wearing of spectacles; variations in hearing are perhaps less obvious but everyone recognizes that they exist – so why do we all think and expect everyone to have the same smell experience? (I wonder if we all have a different experience regarding the sense of touch?)

CASE STORY

On our advanced Diploma course for qualified aromatherapists, we go into olfaction in depth. One lecturer, Dr George Dodd, with a keen interest in olfaction, gave everyone a spill with the same, specific aroma. We all smelled our spill at the same time, then he asked if there was anyone who couldn't smell anything at all; there were 24 in the class and 2 people raised their hands. Then he asked how many liked the smell and 4 people raised their hands. He then asked how many didn't like the smell at all; this time 18 people raised their hands. His next question was – did we know what the smell was? The first few people he asked had no idea, then a couple of people said tentatively, 'It smells like sweat to me' – and they were right!

Does Everyone Benefit from Aromatherapy?

Can aromas affect and benefit people who have no sense of smell?

The name given to the inability to smell aromas is 'anosmia'. One can suffer from total anosmia, when nothing at all can be smelled; specific anosmia, where only some aromas cannot be smelled, or temporary anosmia, which is caused by a heavy cold or chronic sinusitis and returns when the condition returns to normal.

A question you might now ask is 'If a person cannot register a smell, can they still benefit from inhaling essential oils?' When I was talking about inhalation, I said there were two routes the essential oil could travel; one, directly to the brain, the other, via the lungs and hence into the blood stream. Anosmia does not prevent the oils from being absorbed and therefore they will eventually reach the brain via this route.

What about people with a faulty sense of smell?

Not many people suffer from total anosmia, but many people suffer from specific anosmia – often without realizing it. As each cilia at the beginning of the olfactory process has a uniquely shaped depression into which a single aroma molecule can fit, if someone's cilia lack the depressions needed for certain smells, the aroma inhaled will not be recognized. The molecular jigsaw piece which is part of the smell has nowhere to lock into, therefore no signal can be passed to the brain (Price and Price, 1993 p.153). This 'deficiency' is not as obvious as a deficiency in sight, where people realize their sight is failing and can wear glasses to rectify it to some degree. There is no easy means of detecting differences in the ability to smell.

What happens when we are asleep, or have lost our sense of smell?

It seems that humans do react to smells even when asleep (Badia, 1990) and prolonged use of aromas will help to restore a lost sense of smell *(see Case Story below)*. This has also been shown in tests (Holley, 1993). Importantly, smell has been demonstrated to have physiological effects on both normal and anosmic people (Nasel, 1994). Effects of aromas have also been recorded on people in circumstances where the aroma was at such a low level that the people concerned could not detect it (Kirk-Smith & Booth, 1990).

The answer is Yes!

Against the background of the above-mentioned research and my own practical experience, I think it is safe to say that aromas do have an effect on people even:

- when the aroma is not noticeable
- when they are anosmic
- when they are suffering temporary anosmia due to a cold or sinusitis
- when they are asleep.

CASE STORY

One of my clients had suffered from chronic sinusitis for years and his sense of smell had deteriorated over time; he was suffering from prolonged temporary anosmia. After an operation there was no improvement and he found life without being able to smell made him quite miserable at times, especially when returning from work and he could not smell the dinner his wife had cooked for him (she was an excellent cook too!). And worse, he could not taste it either, because smell and taste are very closely linked.

His wife had heard me on the radio and although they lived over 60 miles away, he came to see me. I gave him a 'sandwich' of pressure point massage on his face, supplementing this with SRT (Swiss reflex treatment – 'Swiss' because I 'designed' this successful form of aromatherapy on the feet while on holiday in Switzerland) and then re-doing his face. Two of the oils I used in my synergistic mix were particularly powerful – *Mentha x piperita* (peppermint) and *Eucalyptus globulus* (eucalyptus) yet he could not detect either of them!

He came every Saturday for a treatment, and after the third visit, he thought he could smell something! I put some peppermint onto a spill and held it up to his nose. He let out a delighted yell and said, 'I can smell mint – it's very faint, but I can smell it!' After six months he had recovered his sense of smell sufficiently to be able to appreciate some of the aromas from his wife's cooking – which made life happier for both of them.

I had hoped for some results, however small, as I had just read about recent findings which indicated that in man and animals presenting specific anosmia, the sensitivity to some odours can be restored by repeated exposure to these odours (Wysockietal 1992). In fact, the results were better than I might have expected – with the unexpected side-effect of making their marriage happier!

The Effect of Aromas on our Emotions

We are surrounded nowadays by scents and smells – there is no escape – and unfortunately many of them are synthetic, especially when one looks at household goods and cosmetics. Flavourists spend their working hours trying to imitate flavours, mixing components together in much the same way as a perfumer and, like the perfumer, they are not averse to using synthetics. The thing which amazes both my husband and myself is that some aromatherapists are against using essential oils in waiting rooms, nursing homes and hospitals as they do not wish to 'infringe on personal liberty and choice'. They worry that the person in the next bed may not like the essential oil blend mixed for the person in the first bed. Some will not even use essential oils to aid sleep where the whole ward is suffering from insomnia, for fear of infringing on civil liberty. Essential oils are clean, pure, natural (often the only entirely natural products in the whole building!) and I have found a mixture of their aromas to be only pleasing to all I have met over the last 23 years while teaching and lecturing – thus I find the 'civil liberties' idea in this context difficult to swallow.

I have never heard the same people object to the use of a perfumed cleaning spray in a lift, for example, and I am sure they would object if perfume testing in airports was banned because some passengers may not like that particular aroma. Although there are non-smoking tables in restaurants now, would it enter their heads to think of the people sitting right beside the separation area? Would they object to the smell of new bread emanating from a bakery in a closed-in shopping centre I wonder, in case there are a few people walking along who detest the smell of new bread? Or the use of exotic fragrances at a party to enhance the party feeling (I bet they would not object to that!). Piped music is widely used in restaurants, shops, etc. and so is 'psychedelic' lighting – both can cause distress, yet are widely accepted.

You can see how the thought of all these things is affecting *my* emotions, just because someone is suggesting that the most precious things in my life – helpful to all those with whom I have come into contact – should not be allowed in rooms where there is more than one person! Whenever I have used essential oils in hospital wards, at dinner parties for a relaxing effect or at Christmas parties to give a seasonal aroma, everyone, *everyone* – without exception, – has loved each different aroma. It is not possible for anyone to be adversely affected enough by essential oils for these people to argue about civil liberty!

One of the things influencing my reaction to these people (and therefore my emotions) is the fact that aromas (usually synthetic) are used regularly in places where no-one even thinks of civil liberty – and synthetic smells can actually have an adverse affect on the health – yet we can do nothing about them; there is no choice! One GP (and there are probably more) believes that many of the disorders he comes across during his work are most likely due to commercial air 'fresheners' (Lawson, 1985), which give off unnatural smells, as do the ones given off by most potpourri mixes – which also cause problems to some people.

CASE STORY

Over the years, Len and I have flown to various countries. Len is asthmatic, though his attacks are few and far between now we use essential oils, which enabled him to dispense with his inhaler. There are certain smells, however, which trigger an attack and among these are certain perfumes – not all, so it is obviously particular components in a perfume which aggravate his lungs. (Incidentally, there is not one essential oil in all our 160 which affects him adversely.) At least three times, after boarding an aeroplane, Len has started an attack because a lady near our seat had been trying out perfumes in what was then the Duty-Free, and has had to be moved to another seat – or Club Class if the plane was full.

Another disaster was in a lift which had just been cleaned (with a spray cleaner, we found out later). Just one breath was enough to start him off. Since then, I have to smell inside a lift to check it has not been newly cleaned – and if it has, he takes a deep breath and holds it till we reach our floor. So far, we have not been high enough for him to have to get out before we reach our level! By the way, he cannot go into a shop where potpourri is sold, because the synthetic aromas also bring on his asthma, but at least in this case he has the choice of not going in!

You are no doubt wondering what all this has to do with the emotions. These experiences always provoke in Len the emotion of fear, because once, a particularly strong reaction to something on the farm next to where we were staying in America resulted in a hair-raising drive to the nearest hospital, 20 miles away, and him being in intensive care for three days. I shall never forget it – and for sure, he won't!

We now go prepared for all these eventualities when flying or staying in hotels, taking with us a synergistic mix of:

- basil, which, as a regulator of the nervous system, helps relieve mental strain and anxiety – and
- marjoram, which is not only calming, but is a respiratory tonic too and relaxes bronchial spasm.

We are also never without the oils which help the physical symptoms of bronchial asthma (a mix of basil, eucalyptus, peppermint, lavender and hyssop) – just in case!

I once read a gripping book called *Perfume* by Patrick Süskind; it was the sort of book you cannot put down and was about a perfumer who spent his life searching for one thing to finalize his 'pièce de resistance'. He said that scent was a brother to breath and that human beings could not defend themselves against it. He went on to say:

> scent enters into their very core, goes directly to their hearts, and decides for good and all between affection and contempt, disgust and lust, love and hate. He who rules scent rules the heart of man.
>
> Süskind 1986

Admittedly, he was speaking about all scents, from animals as well as from plants, and I am confident that there is not an essential oil (in current use in aromatherapy, that is) which would conjure up in people disgust or hate. However, it does illustrate how powerfully we can be affected by aromas – of all kinds.

Research has been done which suggested that pleasant odours are likely to influence creative performance, evaluation and personal memories. When compared to unpleasant odours; they:

- enhance creative performance
- generate more positive evaluation of people's words and pictures
- elicit more happy memories (Warren and Warrenburg 1993).

In ancient Greece, writers, philosophers and physicians referred to the influence of aromas on the people. For example, in Homer's *Odyssey,* written before 700BC, the secret of the 'Bouquet of Venus' (which made Aphrodite irresistible) was revealed (Ohloff, 1944 p.VIII). Galen, the Greek physician mentioned earlier, recommended the use of aromatic herbs against hysterical convulsions and considered the fragrance of narcissus (which is a fragrance, not an essential oil) to be 'the food of the soul'. Hyacinth (also a fragrance, not an essential oil) was described by the Greeks as being uplifting and invigorating to a tired mind (Lawless, 1994). So we can see that as well as being used effectively against physical illness, aromatics have been valued for centuries for their effects on the mind, being recommended for their soothing and stimulating properties as well as their ability to alter moods.

CASE STORY

A new friend of mine (who knows little about aromatherapy or essential oils, but who designs gardens and is therefore familiar with fragrant aromas) came round while I was writing this book – and I asked him what effect aromas had on him. This is what he said: 'For me, the impact of aroma or fragrance is as important as any other stimulus in creating a specific mood, feeling or state of mind. It can be most noticeable when moving into an area or room which has a new aroma. Embracing the new fragrance displaces all existing emotional preoccupation and helps change gear to a new state of mind. The power of the olfactory system is such that even slight fragrance can enhance or change the current emotional states.

'My own experience is that vaporizing' (he used the word 'burning' – see next page) 'a cedarwood type of fragrance helps me to concentrate and relax when designing on the computer. Other fragrances have different effects – some of the fragrances I am most familiar with relate to grouping flowers in areas of the landscape to create a specific mood. For instance, the smell of mock orange and certain roses stimulate relaxation, deep inhalation, etc., whereas viburnum, trachelospermum, jasmin and osmanthus together produce a richer, multi-layered smell which is more invigorating.'

What I found most interesting about my garden designer friend's comments was:

- he grouped smells together, thus bearing out my strong belief that one should always use more than one essential oil to create a synergy – the total effect of a synergy is more than the individual effects added together – there is a magical 'extra' dimension when a blend is used
- he had no idea that research had been done in Japan on jasmin where it was found to be, not a relaxing oil, as many of us would assume, but a stimulating one (Torii et al, 1988)!

Incidentally, each essential oil is made up of many different molecules, each with its own shape and size, some evaporating more quickly than others. The individual molecules which evaporate very quickly (and essential oils containing a high proportion of the lighter volatile molecules) are called top notes. Those molecules which evaporate very slowly (and essential oils containing a high proportion of low volatility heavier molecules) are called base notes. Molecules and essential oils which fall somewhere in between these two are called middle notes. Because volatility is most important in designing a lingering perfume, these classifications are given to essential oils and their individual components by the perfume industry.

This difference in volatility is important when using essential oils in a vaporizer or 'burner', as they are frequently and unfortunately called. My friend used the word 'burning', but I prefer to say 'vaporizing'. Burner and burning suggest setting light to something and are associated with acrid smoke. If essential oils are used with the popular nite-light or electric vaporizers, the essential oils are often too close to the heat source. As the lighter and medium molecules of the essential oil vaporize first, the base notes are the last to 'go' and they end up as a somewhat sticky, resinous residue – with a rather unpleasant smell! To minimise this, always put water in the dish first, never letting it dry out.

Conclusion

Several research papers have been published in connection with the effect essential oils can have on the mind, proving beyond doubt that they do have considerable success in this field. Selected references to this kind of research are in this chapter, the rest appearing in some of the other chapters. We have also discovered in this chapter that the quick recognition by the brain of aroma molecules suggests inhalation to be an excellent method to use for emotions needing a 'quick fix', such as sudden shock or over-reaction to a situation, both of which require immediate results.

4 *PNI and Positive Thoughts*

Psychoneuroimmunology (PNI) is a fairly new science – and was not generally known before the 1980s. PNI is the relationship between our emotional state and general health and could be defined as 'the study of how thoughts can influence the brain and directly affect the health of cells in all parts and systems of the body'.

When we understand exactly how this mind/body relationship works, we will be able to appreciate the influence that positive thoughts can have, and how they can counteract negative *health* patterns (which may even have been introduced by our negative *thought* patterns). Once we know how our mind/body interaction affects the health – and appreciate how important is the way we think – we need to go one step further and accept that it is within our power to do something about it. This is where belief in God, Divine Creator or Universal Power, mind dynamics, meditation, yoga and positive thinking enter the picture!

It is difficult to talk about PNI without mentioning the power of positive thought, as they are so closely linked; however, I would like to:

- introduce you to PNI – and how it works
- give the states of mind which influence the health negatively or positively
- describe the different rhythms in the brain at which the mind functions
- reveal how aromas (therefore essential oils) influence brain levels
- specify the brain level most useful for influencing the mind
- explain positive thinking (mind dynamics)
- show how you can practise positive thinking successfully yourself.

Introduction

All forms of human functioning are involved in energy. The energy patterns given off by the human body (which can be shown by Kirlian photography) are different in health and disease and are significantly influenced by mental processes and emotional states. A great number of people believe, unfortunately, that their whole existence is confined simply to the physical aspects of their body; what they do not realize is that they are exploring and living only *one fifth of their potential*. They cannot appreciate 'the other four fifths of who they are and the part the "higher levels" play in their complete self' (Bennett, 1989).

If we are able understand how PNI and positive thoughts can affect our lives, we will be able more easily to accept the above, which at first glance seems almost bizarre. Let's look at the word itself. If we split up the word psycho – neuro – immun – ology, it tells us exactly what is involved: the study *(ology)* of the mind *(psyche)*, the nervous system *(neuro)* and the immune system *(immun)*.

The Immune System

It is only in the last few decades that the immune system has become as much a part of anatomy as the nine systems which have been known for centuries (skeletal, muscular, circulatory – cardiovascular, lymphatic, digestive, excretory, glandular, reproductive and nervous). The immune system is the body's defence against disease: when a child is immunized against catching an unwanted disease in future years, the body produces antibodies to fight (successfully) against the minute injection of that disease. These antibodies stay within the human system and prevent the disease taking hold, should the child be exposed to it in the future; in other words, the injection has strengthened the immune system.

If we are under severe stress or suffering from a long-standing illness, the immune system becomes weakened and is unable to produce enough antibodies to protect us from every germ which appears on the scene; because of stress and the weakened immune system, we become prone to disease.

The questions we would all like answered are:

- How can the way we think have such an enormous influence on our immune system and our health generally (physically, emotionally and spiritually)?
- What makes the interaction of body, mind and spirit have such a great influence on whether we are successful and healthy, or unhappy and in ill-health?
- Can a pessimistic outlook really influence our immune system directly?

The physical basis of psychoneuroimmunology is explained below, but the wonder of it, the amazing connection between the psychological and physical effects, is difficult to grasp.

The cardiovascular, nervous and immune systems, together with the brain (mind), have all been researched independently, and in the last few years, psychologists, neuroscientists and immunologists working together discovered a definite link between these systems, which led to the new discipline psychoneuroimmunology.

In her book *Minding the body, mending the mind*, Joan Borysenko explains that a group of hormonal messengers called neuropeptides are produced by the brain, the immune system and also by nerve cells in various other organs. The areas of the brain which control the emotions are particularly well supplied with receptors for these neuropeptides and the brain also has receptor sites for two other chemicals, which are produced only by the immune system. This gives us a remarkable 'two-way communication system linking the mind, the immune system, and potentially all other systems, a pathway through which our emotions – our hopes and fears – can affect the body's ability to defend itself' (Borysenko, 1987).

In the last ten to fifteen years:

> ... we have had a major breakthrough in the study of mind-body connections. We have learned that there are direct connections between the brain, the nervous system, the glands that produce our hormones and the immune system itself.
>
> Wood, 1990 p.119

States of Mind which Influence Health

The significance of the above is overwhelming – to think that the mind, the nervous system and the immune system are not separate entities, as previously thought, but actually communicate with each other, affecting the health, for good or bad, depending partly on what goes on in our mind. This interaction 'appears to affect behaviour, emotion and mood, as well as physical performance' (Wingate & Wingate, 1988). When the body is fighting infection, for example, this intercommunication keeps the brain informed about what is happening in the body, and when we are suffering severe stress, depression or destructive emotions such as anguish, depression, desolation, grief, heartache, pain and worry, this same intercommunication suppresses the ability of the immune system to destroy the bacteria causing the infection, which may result in illness. The severity of the illness depends on how long the state of mind or emotion has been part of one's life, which group it falls into and, of course, its intensity.

Psychosomatic (mind/body) medicine arises from the mind having power over the body (see Case Story, p.30). What we believe becomes the biology of our body, that is, the mind of the sufferer creates its own scene for either a happy outcome of a distressful situation or the continuation/worsening of the same situation. Our thoughts and emotions (and therefore the words we speak) determine whether our body cells decide to take either a healthy path or a diseased one. Positive emotions have a beneficial physiological effect and negative emotions have a pathological (relating to or causing disease) effect.

CASE STORY

When I was a teenager, one of my favourite aunts died. She and Uncle Wilton had no children and lived only for each other. When Auntie Maidie died, my uncle, who was in perfect health, lost all interest in life, repeating all the time that he just wanted to die, to be with her. The family tried to comfort him, but in three months he too died. The doctor told the family there was no reason at all for his death and that, in his opinion, he had died of a broken heart. All these years later, I can see how this could have happened.

Various researchers who have examined the link between emotions and illness have found a strong association between depression, grief, and suppression of the immune system. Regarding mourners at funerals, for example, even 100 years ago it was recognized that 'the depression of spirits at these melancholy occasions ... disposes them to some of the worst effects of the chills' (Editorial: *British Medical Journal*, 1884).

Psychologists who have studied the lives of cancer patients found that many had experienced depression prior to the development of the cancer, some due to grieving for their husband or wife, others following their child being diagnosed with leukaemia (Gerber, 1988).

CASE STORY

A colleague and friend of mine lost her only daughter at the age of 18 months. The grieving process lasted several years, Sonia taking every opportunity to remember her daughter – and re-live her grief. Eventually, after seven years, she developed cancer, and even at the time, the doctors were not averse to considering the possibility of it being connected with her grief. The prognosis was very poor, but she was determined to pull through. The major part of her problem was that she was unable to forgive herself for the events which had led up to her daughter's death. She could not accept that there was nothing that she could have done differently at the time. The start of her healing process was realizing this and letting go of the self-recrimination.

Four months later, Sonia trained to be an aromatherapist because she wanted to understand the human body and its workings, and she never again wanted to be in the position of not recognizing when someone was ill. She later studied positive thinking and through her positive thoughts and attitude, using positive imaging and positive visualization, she was eventually, after two to three years, clear of her cancer. She had learned, with the help of essential oils (frankincense and rose otto in lime blossom macerated carrier oil, which she called 'a hug in a bottle' – delightful!), to let go of the past and accept that her grieving would never bring her daughter back and, in fact, had only resulted in her living a life of continual regret, trying unsuccessfully to suppress her feelings, for her husband's sake. Now that she has come to terms with, and accepted, the loss of her daughter, she has found a new happiness – and a strengthened marriage.

> Excess of grief for the dead is madness: for it is an injury to the living and the dead know it not.
>
> Xenophon

Psychoneuroimmunology is the science which has made us understand to some extent that 'we are what we think', proving that negative thoughts and emotions are self-inflicted wounds which effectively close down the immune system, leaving the body open to a wide range of disease processes. It becomes clear therefore that the immune system is under the influence of mental and emotional experiences and *we* are at the helm; our thoughts are the 'managing director' of the body and the body faithfully reproduces the wishes dictated by our mind processes. All destructive emotions will eventually express themselves through the body in a negative way, and emotions like anger, hate, jealousy, envy, guilt and greed (even lack of self-love and/or -confidence) – as well as fear and grief – will influence the immune system and predispose us towards health breakdown.

It is interesting, but sad, that many actors who repeatedly play the lead in Shakespeare's *Macbeth* and singers of depressing songs tend to become ill (because their minds are continually sending negative commands to the immune system). I have also noticed that many people who dress themselves completely and continuously in black (for which fashion and sometimes the adulation of pop stars is largely responsible), without the relief of a bright scarf, blouse, tie or shirt, often have a morose outlook on life and tend to express aggressive, negative and destructive thoughts.

Conversely, productive, happy and positive thoughts (and happy colours!) exert a positive influence on the behaviour of body cells, resulting in an improvement in both health (even if there is no disease) and well-being. Norman Cousins found that laughter is an excellent aid to recovery from a depressing disease, using it himself when he was unable to find relief through allopathic drugs. He shut himself in a room with some Charlie Chaplin videos – and laughed his way back to health! (Cousins, 1979)

CASE STORY

I practise something similar myself if ever I am feeling a bit 'down' (it doesn't happen very often, thank goodness!) and it certainly helps to dispel any unhappy or miserable thoughts I may have. The first time I tried it was when I was driving to work on a dark, rainy day in lots of traffic, with all the things I had to do when I got there spinning through my mind. I stretched my mouth into a big 'smile', even though I was not feeling in the least like smiling. After a couple of minutes of keeping my mouth stretched (from ear to ear), I realized I was no longer depressed or miserable, but more like my normal self. The smile had become real, and by the time I reached work, ten minutes later, I felt quite cheerful! The change in my emotional well-being also benefited those with whom I came into contact, as my words were said with a smile, rather than a straight face, or perhaps even a frown! After that, I practised it every time I felt dejected, irritable or sad – and it worked *every* time. It will naturally not rectify the *reason* why one is depressed, angry or jealous, but it certainly alters the frame of mind and the emotion experienced; certainly those to whom I have recommended trying it have been astonished at their success.

This exercise is excellent whenever you have thoughts about yourself or other people which seem destructive or negative. It is also a sound introduction to a positive thinking session, so do try it! Using a forced smile is a conscious activity to start the process of healing (body, mind or spirit). This is positivity in action and takes effort to accomplish. On the contrary, the opposite effect takes no effort at all; you can take a backward step in health – unconsciously – without even trying. Which would you prefer? The effort is well worth while!

CASE STORY

I have a friend who, whenever I ask how she is (as one does), always answers without fail 'tired'. Admittedly, she has three young children, two at school (one full time and one three mornings a week) but she doesn't go to work, and I have many friends (with two to four children) who go to work full time and whose reply when I ask the same question is 'fine, thanks!' Angela is a lovely girl and appears to be both healthy and happily married and I would love to persuade her to realize that the more she says she is tired, the more tired she is going to be – and that her health will suffer as a result. Unfortunately, she has no faith in such possibilities. Incidentally, a survey in America in the 1970s revealed that the most powerful reason for fatigue was not physical, but psychological. People who were depressed or anxious were seven times more likely to feel tired than those without emotional problems (Chen, 1986).

Angela is certainly not depressed, but she is always anxious. For example, when one of the children falls over, she assumes he or she may have broken a bone; if one knocks his head against something hard, she worries that the eye (or perhaps even the brain!) will be affected and she and her husband dash off to the doctor. Angela's case is not a serious one; however, it is enough to serve as an example of how a state of mind can cause physical tiredness.

Brain Rhythms

When under severe stress or suffering from a long-standing or debilitating illness, the brain is in a different rhythm from when we are completely at peace. It has four levels of consciousness, at different frequencies: the one we live in daily is the 'Beta level' and is the level which operates at the highest (or fastest) frequency, the top mark of which is around 25 Hertz. Each level operates at a progressively slower rate, Delta functioning at the slowest frequency of all four, at its lowest, a mere 4 Hertz or less.

- *Beta level* has the highest frequency of the four levels, around 14–25 Hz, and all adults think at this level when they are awake. The higher the level, the more wide awake and alert we are – but when agitated or under stress, we function very near the top end of the scale. At Beta level we are physically in control of our five senses; we can see, touch, taste, hear and smell – but we are limited in time and space to the here and now. At this level, we are in a critical, judgemental mode.
- *Alpha level* is at 8–13 Hz and is the level which adults reach when they are very, very relaxed. When we first wake in the morning we

are automatically at Alpha level and dreams usually take place at this level. We can also make a better impression on our brain at this level; it is the most impressionable for creative work and accepts more easily any visualization we may have. Here, we see, touch, hear, smell and taste *inside the mind;* we can see pictures of where we spent our holidays, smell the sea and hear the waves – all inside our mind; at this level, time and space vanish. At this level, we are in a creative mode.

During the day, we continually slip in and out of the Alpha and Beta levels.

I carry out all my mind dynamics and positive thinking at Alpha level, the course I attended having taught us how to reach this state of relaxation and use it to our best advantage.

Children up to about seven years old are in Alpha level most of the time. You have probably noticed that children are very imaginative: they play games with an imaginary friend; they talk to their toys, who give them answers back, etc. Because children live in Alpha they are more receptive to the influences around them, which is why the poem near the beginning of Chapter 2 is so true. Parents should be very careful of how they act and what they say in front of children, as each situation is a reality to a child – they take in more than one thinks and remember much more than one wants them to.

- *Theta level* has a frequency of 4–7 Hz; the waves are fairly irregular and we are never at this level in our conscious state. Sleep is deepest in the early stages of the sleep cycle and this deep sleep takes place at Theta level. Children occasionally reach this brain wave level, especially in the first couple of years of life. Although adults are never in this level when awake, it is possible to reach it when practising positive thinking, meditation or yoga. Those who can attain it can control physical pain and bleeding, although to reach this level by yourself, you would need to attend a mind dynamics course. Theta level can also take effect under hypnosis.
- *Delta level* has a frequency of only 4 Hz or less. Babies still in the womb are at a Delta level of consciousness, and for the first few days after birth they fluctuate between all four brain rhythms. For the next few weeks they are mostly in Delta, moving gradually

into Theta level, and up to the age of seven spend most of their time in the Alpha level of the brain; they are not fully in the Beta level until the age of about 12–14. Delta level never occurs in adults – except perhaps during *very* deep sleep (especially if sedated) and also under an anaesthetic.

Primitive man lived mostly in the lower three levels and was delighted when he began to use his Beta level more; this is progress or civilization (evolution), and man has made use of this Beta level more and more as each century has passed. However, just as our sense of smell has diminished since we no longer have to hunt our own food, so the natural use of the Alpha level has diminished also. We now live in a more aggressive world which induces stress, and we need to recover our ability to live in calm and peace of mind (Everett, 1973).

The Effect of Aromas on Brain Levels

Recent studies have been done on how aromatic substances exert their action on the mind and body through inhalation, that is, their effect on the four different levels of brain activity.

An American, John Steele, carried out some experiments to discover the effects of several essential oils and absolutes on the various brain levels. He found that:

- basil, rosemary, black pepper and cardamom induced Beta-predominant patterns, which are associated with aroused attention and alertness
- orange blossom, jasmine and rose (not essential oils, but absolutes, which are heavier and sweeter) induced a variety of lower levels of brain activity, Alpha indicating a quietening of mental chatter and Theta and Delta indicating the mind going into reverie, with intuitive flashes (Steele, 1984).

Professor Torii, in Japan, carried out studies to determine whether certain aromas were stimulant, sedative or neutral. His results, which were dependent on the person's individual perception and experience of the oils presented, showed that:

- lavender was sedative
- jasmine was stimulant
- geranium and rosewood were either sedative or stimulant (Torii, 1988).

The writer, Michel Eyquem de Montaigne, born 1533 and one-time Mayor of Bordeaux, invented the literary form of the essay: in 1580, his 'Essay on Smell' was published and included the following words:

> Physicians might ... make greater use of scents than they do, for I have often noticed that they cause changes in me, and act on my spirits ... which makes me agree with the theory that the introduction of incense and perfume into the churches ... was for the purpose of raising our spirits, and of exciting and purifying our senses, the better to fit us for contemplation.

Using Alpha Level to Direct the Mind

The brain-wave level most useful for influencing the mind – and therefore our emotions – is the second level of consciousness, the Alpha brain rhythm. At this rhythm or level we are in a completely relaxed and open frame of mind, where brain activity is reduced, leaving space for 'organized' thoughts to take precedence. At this level there is scope for visualization (which the Bristol Cancer Help Centre, among others, encourage their patients to practise), for developing and creating new projects and designs, for meditation and prayer – and to put positive thoughts into action.

If we can trigger the Alpha rhythm of the brain, we can become a more effective person, with extra power to become more inspired and even find our sixth sense. Some people, for example Beethoven, are inspired intuitively or by accident; most of us have to be taught how to do it. We all have the same 'equipment', but have to learn how to use it – how to make it work for us – and we all have different talents waiting to be brought to the fore (if they are not already evident).

There are various methods by which one can reach this level of mind, including meditation, mind dynamics, music, prayer and yoga.

We are naturally in this deep state of relaxation first thing in the morning, just as we wake up, which is the time when I both pray and practise my positive thinking. Also, the research above confirms that sedative essential oils, such as Roman chamomile, bitter orange, bergamot, lavender and melissa could be put to good use to induce the brain to drop into Alpha level and more easily accept your positive thoughts and make imagery and viualization effortless.

There is not the space in this book to devote to mind dynamics because I could write a book on this subject alone; perhaps I will one day! It needs a book to itself in order to learn thoroughly the methods by which one can, at any time of day, descend not only to Alpha level, but even to Theta level of brain waves; in Alpha alone we can not only achieve physical and mental health and well-being for ourselves (plus goals we may aspire to in life), but also make a positive impression on the health and well-being of others. However, no doubt many readers can already reach their Alpha level by either prayer and faith in God, meditation, yoga, or perhaps mind dynamics; if you find it difficult, simply use sedative and relaxing essential oils. It is then just a matter of taking responsibility for your own life and health, and with a belief in the power of positive thinking you can change your life!

Incidentally, research has just been completed by the British Psychological Society on 474 students to discover if there was any correlation between personal prayer and well-being (anxiety, depression and self-esteem). The results were reported on the radio and showed that those who prayed were considerably happier than those who did not (Maltby *et al*, 1999).

Positive Thinking

Positive thoughts, repeated over and over again, can achieve physical and mental well-being without using meditation, mind dynamics or yoga. The important thing is to repeat your thoughts as often as you can – out loud, in writing, by singing – *every* day. I was first introduced to the power of positive thinking through a book of my father's (with that as its title) written by Norman Vincent Peale in 1953 and reprinted 26 times by 1992. In his first chapter, he says:

Believe in yourself! Have faith in your abilities! Without humble but reasonable confidence in your own powers you cannot be successful or happy ... self-confidence leads to self-realisation and successful achievement.

Peale 1992

One of the main affirmations he gave people was one I say myself now every day – 'I can do everything through Him, who gives me strength' (Philippians 4:13). A few years later, I was given Anne Infante's affirmations cassette *(see page 74)* by a friend and I play that every morning either in the car going to work, or in the garage, where my husband I play table tennis for half an hour each morning. Both the book and the cassette have certainly had amazing and wonderful effects on my own life.

Several people have written books involving positive thinking (or other names meaning the same thing) and because it is known to have such a major influence on how we live our lives, it is often included in books which are concerned either with different complementary disciplines, lack of self-confidence or success in business.

If people were asked a few simple questions on how they viewed life, the results would be varied. Clive Wood tells of an experiment carried out to discover how many people were 'life affirmers' and how many were what he calls 'life deniers'. The results were most interesting, the main features he gleaned from analysing the replies to his set of questions being as follows:

- life affirmers displayed enthusiasm, sociability, unselfishness, happiness, satisfaction with life, optimism and good physical health
- life deniers displayed unsociability, selfishness, emotional instability, depression, pessimism, lack of drive and dissatisfaction with life (Wood, 1990 pp.21–3).

Life affirmers are either natural positive thinkers – or have practised it successfully; life deniers are definitely in need of positive thinking lessons! It would be a good idea if lessons in positive thinking were given at school, as these could help people to benefit from all aspects of life, giving them the opportunity to change those they may not like. It may also reduce the number and/or frequency of destructive emotions which could show themselves in our lives, thus benefiting those around us as well.

We need to practise positive thinking to ensure that destructive emotions never 'get the better' of us – and therefore do not affect our health adversely. With continuous practice you will discover that not only can you improve your health, but you can more or less achieve whatever you desire by determination – *love* and *faith*. People often refer to an excellent book on their favourite subject as their 'bible'; this is because the Holy Bible itself contains so many home truths and aids to a successful life. I have already quoted 1 Corinthians 13 on the subject of love in Chapter 1; here are two on faith:

> Faith is being sure of what we hope for and certain of what we do not see.
>
> Hebrews 11:1

> If you do not stand firm in your faith, you will not stand at all.
>
> Isaiah 7:9

When you read the case story below, I am sure you will appreciate that positive thinking is inescapably linked with PNI.

When I went on my mind dynamics course I was not sure what I wanted to learn from it. We were told it would be a great help in developing our businesses and would keep us in good health, but I never dreamed that it would change my life completely! We were asked on the first day what we would like to change about ourselves – and were shown exactly how to do it. We were told that our measure of success would depend on our own strength of thought and our belief that it *was* possible to achieve the aspects in our lives that we wanted to change for the better.

CASE STORY

When I reached the age of 30, I was almost 'waiting' for arthritis to develop in my hands. It had started this way and at this age with my mother and we had been told it was hereditary. Sure enough, shortly after my 30th birthday, I found I could not squeeze out the dishcloth tightly (just like my mother!), then my fingers began to hurt and swell, also the bone at the base of my thumb became painful and enlarged. Luckily for me, when I was 40, by which time my joints were quite swollen and stiff, I was persuaded to go on a mind dynamics course (nothing to with my arthritis – why I went is yet another story!).

On the course we were told we could get rid of bad habits like smoking, cure problems like constipation, insomnia and other health problems simply by using our minds. The idea was incredible and I became more and more fascinated as the week progressed. Before the end of the week, I was able to sleep the whole night through (and later threw away my tablets); I cured myself of constipation, from which I had suffered since the age of 14 (after four weeks I was – and am still – regular as clockwork); best of all, I was shown how to get rid of the arthritis! This took a little longer than the other two to show results, but as well as daily visualization in my Alpha level workshop, I talked firmly to my hands at Beta level and told them I was *not* going to have arthritis.

I suddenly realized, when I had been home only about 9 months, that I couldn't remember when I last had pain in my fingers or thumbs – and I was squeezing out cloths tightly! That was 27 years ago, and although my joints have retained their 'funny', lumpy shape, I am, thanks to mind dynamics and positive thoughts, free of the arthritis and pain, which is the most important thing.

Some of the things people on the mind dynamics course said about their lives were:

• Smoking is just a habit with me/I can't stop myself smoking – I wish I could
• I'll never have any money to go on holiday/buy a new car, etc.
• I hate my job, but I suppose I'll be there the rest of my life like my father
• I can't sleep without sleeping tablets
• I bet I get arthritis like my mother
• I'll always be fat – no diet works for me

- My sister has a much better life than me
- I wish I were as successful as ... (neighbour, friend, etc).

All these expressions are negative – very negative. The problem is that our minds are very obedient – they do exactly what they are told (remember the links and interconnections between the emotions, body and brain?)! If we continually say to ourselves, day after day, 'I am so fat', we will always be fat! It's as simple as that. The mind is conditioned to do what its owner believes and/or instructs it to do, whether these instructions are positive or negative. The results are exactly like training a dog; a well-trained dog does exactly as it has been taught, even if it is to attack and bite people, like a police dog.

CASE STORY

A minister friend of mine, who was very overweight (18½ stone – mostly in front!), decided to lose weight as a way of earning money for our church. He asked sponsors for £1 a pound and everyone was happy to do this as they didn't think he would be able to lose too much in the time stated (six months) because he loves his food and he is not a tall man to start with.

Bob told me that because he had decided to do it, sticking to the diet was part of the decision. He did so well in the first few weeks, a ceiling had to be put on the amount of money people would have to pay. At the end of the allotted time (Christmas), he had lost 6½ stone, attaining an almost unbelievable, but much more attractive, weight of 12 stone.

He told me 'change happens because we want it to – I'm an experienced expert!'

If we can consciously change our thinking and train our minds to carry out what we really want instead of repeatedly complaining about how we are, we could turn all these 'miseries' into happinesses. All we have to do is to believe in our capability to change our thinking. What we *should* be saying, day after day, is:

- It is easy for me to give up smoking; I *feel* much better without cigarettes

- I am wealthy; I have plenty of money; I am going to the Azores next year; I can afford a car
- I can easily get a job I love doing
- I can sleep without sleeping tablets
- I refuse to have arthritis (or whatever)
- I am slim and beautiful – I can stick to any diet
- I am successful in my business and run it well
- I love my sister.

I cannot emphasize enough that *we are what we think*; if we continually say positive things to ourselves, they *will* come to pass, but it needs hard work and determination – and belief in the method.

CASE STORY

When Len and I started our own business, 29 years ago, we had a 90 per cent mortgage on our house. We had only £100 in the bank – for emergencies. After going on the mind dynamics course again, with Len, I persuaded him to leave the job he hated, and train as a trichologist, which would be helpful to me as a hairdresser (I had a tiny shop in the village where we lived). Our earning capacity was now rather low to maintain the mortgage and two growing children, so we decided we should open a hairdressing and beauty salon in a nearby town, with a trichology clinic, sauna and solarium (the machine before sun beds were invented).

The estate agent was a client of mine and she found us ideal premises. It was more than we could afford, so we worked every day on our mind dynamics, determined that we would have it and work together. We were still worried about the risk we would be taking – the building needed a lot of work doing to it. A week later, the agent returned to say that the owners would accept an offer below the asking price if we could begin negotiations right away. She could see that we were suffering emotions of fear and doubt, yet wanting to say 'yes', and she said firmly: 'Give me your cheque for £100 now and we'll work something out later'! ... So we did!

We worked like Trojans for three months and set our opening date for the second Monday in September. I asked the editor of the local newspaper to open The Birch Twig, as we called it, and in return we would give her our 'Top to Toe' treatment (sauna, solarium, massage, facial and hair cut). Two weeks before opening, I wrote to every doctor and nurse in the area, inviting them to the opening, where they would be offered a tour round, a soft drink and some snacks.

The week before, the carpet for the stairs had still not arrived and neither had the sauna; we really needed our mind dynamics to keep us going! The sauna arrived on the Friday, and we went to fetch the carpet ourselves that afternoon, as the delivery date would be too late. I had asked my sister if I could borrow a wonderful collage she had made to put on the wall behind the buffet and she arrived with it on the Saturday afternoon. We eagerly showed her round, really proud of ourselves!

After looking at the shop, kitchen and coffee bar, we mounted the stairs; she looked at the half-laid carpet and unhung curtains – and we continued up to the next floor to see the slendertone machine, the solarium and the half-assembled sauna (such things as these were hardly known then, by the way). My sister then spoke saying, in a voice which set my heart thumping, 'Do you think you'll finish in time?' and continuing in a 'beyond belief' kind of voice, 'Do you think anyone will come?'

I will never *ever* forget that moment. Suddenly we panicked. We finished everything about midday on Sunday, absolutely shattered and anxious; whatever would we do if we had no customers? We prepared the food for the buffet, then lay in bed (we couldn't sleep) using our mind dynamics to visualize lots of people coming through the door the next day. We rose at 6 o'clock to make the sandwiches – and set off – to what?

About 27 people came to the opening; no doctors, but a few doctors' wives came with their friends, and half a dozen or so other people, who had read about it in the paper. Having written about 100 letters and worked really hard in our workshops, we were fearful of what would happen now … However, after an introduction and an escorted tour, we gave them our price list and, during the buffet, *eight* people made appointments for a series of slendertone treatments, which paid the wages, for *two* weeks, of *both* girls we had employed the week before!

In this story, you will recognize the difference between negative and positive thoughts and how they affect the mind. People who always think the worst attract negative happenings; not only that, but it always pays to go one stage further than 'looking on the bright side' and consciously visualize how you want your life, your health and your *attitude* to life to be. Without my own positive thoughts, my sister's negativity could have had a disastrous effect on the success of that opening day – and indeed, on our whole future!

CASE STORY

As a sequel to the story above, I must tell you that on Fridays I quickly became solidly booked with hair appointments. This meant that occasionally, and especially if a customer was late, I had to keep someone waiting. However, if I remembered on Friday mornings to include (in my mind dynamics, which I practised every morning before getting up) visualizing myself doing people's hair at really high speed, one after the other, I never kept anyone waiting, however busy the day. The amazing thing is that if, for some reason, I forgot the visualization, I *always* got a bit behind (even with the same regulars). I soon learned not to forget!

Practising Positive Thinking

About ten years after this experience, a former aromatherapy student of mine spoke at one of our Open Days on positive thinking. On that day I learned that although thoughts are tremendously powerful, words are even more powerful – up to ten times as powerful. Thoughts, unspoken, affect only ourselves, whereas the spoken word can delight, terrify, influence, harm, cheer or amuse other people. This is why it is always best to think – and pause – before we speak; 'Speak in haste – repent at leisure'; this can cause us more pain or anxiety than if we considered our words before speaking them:

God created a world by the word; you create a little world by your words. God's world was beautiful until the words of man made it as it is today ... Words paint a picture of you to the world; it may be beautiful, it may be ugly, ... and if you were to see its colour, you would hang your head very low when you saw the ugliness of the colour that comes from the words you have said ... *However*, if you say a word in kindness and love, ... it returns to you in the love that is given in exchange *(the word in italics is mine)*

Dr Lascelles

In 1986 I was given the cassette I mentioned on page 67, which necessitated singing out loud; this cassette has enabled me to reinforce my mind dynamics in a happy, joyful way. It opens with these words:

We use affirmations to change our old negative thought patterns to new positive abundant thoughts that work for our good. It's been said that we are the sum total of our thoughts, so if we don't like the way we are, it's essential to change the way we think. Affirmations are a positive, fun way to begin.

Here are some simple rules:

- Watch what you say; if you find yourself using negative, hopeless words to describe yourself, your life or those around you, stop right there and change the thought to a positive one. Remember, we become what we think about every day.
- Affirmations work to the degree that you are willing to put energy into them, so don't mumble them down in your boots; energize them, say them, sing them out loud, revel in them, express them joyfully and with conviction. It doesn't matter if you don't believe them at first; when you see them begin to work for you, you'll be convinced.
- Be persistent. You have spent many years becoming the way you are; you've worked faithfully on yourself since childhood. Changing all that hard work isn't likely to be an overnight job, but remember the old saying – if you won't be beat, you can't be beat. Persistence does pay off, with wonderful results. Give yourself half an hour every day of positive affirmations and say them again as you go to sleep.

I wish you a wonderful, positive, happy, healthy and successful life – and now on with the singing!

Infante, 1986

I am going to quote the words from some of the songs because I
believe they may be able to help you as they helped me – I am only
sorry you will not be able to hear the music as you read them – but
the words alone can help and, hopefully, the tape is still available
should you wish to send for it. The following, together with its tune,
is my favourite:

> I love life and life loves me, I love life and life loves me
> I love life and life loves me – and life and I agree.
> And life and I agree, and life and I agree
> And life and I agree, and life and I agree
> And life and I agree, and life and I agree
> And life and I agree – we are in harmony

Note the repetition, which is so important for positive thinking.
There are five further verses, each substituting another attribute for
'life': health, peace, wealth, joy and love. You can add other verses
(as you haven't got the music) for whatever attributes you want for
yourself. If it is your health you want to improve, you can say (out
loud!) one of the verses from another song:

> I believe in perfect health; I believe in perfect health
> I believe in perfect health, perfect health in my life today.

Then the words of yet another of her songs will become real for you:

> Every day and in every way, I'm getting better and better and
> better.

You can repeat this one too with different words – 'younger',
'richer', 'stronger', etc.

A few of the verses from one of the songs are relevant to the emotions we are discussing and I cannot close the chapter without giving
them to you:

grief:
I relax, I release, I let go all grief
I relax, I release, I always find relief

fear:
I relax, I release, I let go all fear
I relax, I release, I know my good is near

anger:
I relax, I release, I let go all anger
I relax, I release, my joy will last much longer

There are more, which are relevant to other emotions or states of mind in which we may find ourselves:

greed:
I relax, I release, I let go all greed
I relax, I release, for I have all I need

confusion:
I relax, I release, I let go confusion
I relax, I release, and recognize illusion

lies:
I relax, I release, I let go all lies
I relax, I release, my words are calm and wise

resentment:
I relax, I release, I let go resentment
I relax, I release, and I'm filled with contentment

the past:
I relax, I release, I let go the past
I relax, I release, my happiness will last

sorrow:
I relax, I release, I let go all sorrow
I relax, I release, I'll have a bright tomorrow

mistakes:
I relax, I release, I let go mistakes
I relax, I release, for I've got what it takes

hate:
I relax, I release, I let go all hate
I relax, I release, I know my life is great

pain:
I relax, I release, I let go all pain
I relax, I release, I'm in good health again

disease:
I relax, I release, I let go disease
I relax, I release, I'm healthy as I please

The first song starts 'I walk forward confidently' and if you can do that, you are sure to walk forward 'to health and happiness'! Thank you, Anne Infante!

Conclusion

Great progress has been made in our knowledge of the interaction between the mind, emotions, nervous system and immune system, and there is growing recognition of their combined impact on general health. Essential oils have an effect on everyone and play an important role in bringing about a state of relaxation, which favourably affects healing (Price & Price, 1999).

Both orthodox and complementary medicine now acknowledge (perhaps on account of the enormous amount of research which has been done on the subject) that a positive mental attitude is important in any attempt to recover from ill-health.

It is equally invaluable in recovering from damaged and hurt emotions. Norman Cousins was right when he said that drugs are not always necessary – but belief always is. Belief and trust in the power of God or Universal Power, belief in the power of meditation, belief in the power of yoga – one must have faith of some kind. It is essential – *vital* – to enable the body and mind together to act every single day, through our thoughts, to promote our own good, our own health, our own well-being. Faith can move mountains – and the mountains we build for ourselves in our own minds are no exception.

5 Selecting Essential Oils for the Emotions

When aromatherapy first came to the UK, its main (some would say its only) concern was to treat stress. No claims were made to treat specific health conditions, but because aromatherapy is a holistic discipline, therapists indirectly treated the presenting symptoms by treating the stress itself. Many essential oils have a relaxing and beneficial action on both mild and severe stress, and a competent aromatherapist would choose, from these oils, those which would also benefit the symptoms showing themselves – not forgetting the emotional aspect if, for instance, stress is making the client irritable or frightened. If it is an emotion that is *causing* the stress, such as grief, worry, deep-seated anger and so on, the choice will be made from those in the stress-relieving list which will have a positive and beneficial effect on those emotions *(see Chapter 7)*. In hospitals, essential oils have been found to be capable of relieving stress, raising the spirits, strengthening and revitalizing the mind and bringing comfort to the body by easing some of the distressing effects of the illness being suffered (Price & Price, 1999 p.242).

In allopathic medicine, treatment of any kind is mostly aimed specifically at the symptom or organ giving a problem. In aromatherapy, which has, like other complementary therapies, a holistic approach, the whole person is considered – to discover, if possible, the *cause* behind the symptoms experienced and to treat that. It may be found that there is an ongoing stressful situation (problems at work, divorce, environment) – or perhaps something in life has a depressive element in it – such as bereavement or a failing business. It may be that deep-seated anger or grief is revealed.

An aromatherapist would therefore select essential oils *firstly* to benefit the mental state of the person rather than the isolated symptoms. As I said previously, each essential oil is capable of various effects, these effects depending on the properties of the individual oil – that is, whether it is analgesic, anti-inflammatory, decongestant, etc. While relaxing or uplifting the state of mind, and research confirms that this can be done with essential oils (Buchbauer *et al*, 1993), the body can also receive help from other attributes the oil may possess, such as the relief of muscle pain and digestive problems.

My husband compares the effects of allopathic medicine and essential oils to the effects of two kinds of guns:

- allopathic medicine uses a rifle, which fires one bullet (i.e. one drug) at a time at the target – in this case, one specific symptom. Each drug consists of one type of molecule only
- aromatherapy uses a shotgun, which sprays a myriad of pieces of lead shot (i.e. essential oil properties) at a time at the target – in this case the whole body. Each essential oil contains hundreds of different molecules.

Over the years, the more involved (obsessed might be a better word!) I became with essential oils the more I wanted 'proof' of their effects. Some of the physical properties have been found traditionally (and in a few instances proved by research) to have some of the effects claimed and I prefer to recommend only these, resisting the temptation to give other properties sometimes accredited to them. As far as their effect on disturbed emotions is concerned, there is very little evidence as yet – even anecdotal – so how have I been able to select beneficial oils with confidence?

I decided that the best way to explain how essential oils can affect the emotions would be to apply the same principles employed for helping physical problems. After all, the mind has a tremendous effect on the body, and as some essential oils have been shown to relax and others to uplift, there is every reason to suppose that analgesic oils will relieve the pain of grief, anti-inflammatory oils will dampen the inflammation of anger, and so on.

> Went home to take some fennouillet *(old English for fennel water)*, I was so sick of him.
>
> Swift

Pliny (AD 23–79) recommended fennel not only for the physical eye-sight, but also for the second sight, to see clearly the beauty of nature. He said also that the fennel plant was loved by serpents because it aided them to slough off their old skins and thus rejuvenate themselves.

Nevertheless, I prefer to say that certain oils *may* help this or that emotion, rather than saying they *will* help. Every person is an individual; each one of us has his/her own characteristics, personality and beliefs which make up the whole person, influencing how and what we think – and how we behave. We even experience emotions and bear pain according to our individual characteristics; we cannot be categorized and therefore each of us may react differently. A perfect example of our individuality is in our faces; yes, we all have two eyes, a nose and a mouth, but how often, from the billions of people in the world, do you meet anyone who looks *exactly* like you?

Despite the fact that we are all different, I have confidence in the *reasons* behind my approach, which I have found to work very well for my clients (and my students' clients) over the years. Because I believe the physical properties of essential oils can have an influence on emotional experiences, this relationship is fully explained below:

Analgesic

Many essential oils have pain-killing properties – to different degrees and for different systems of the body, some relieving pain in joints and muscles, as in arthritis, others seeming more efficient for headaches. There seems to be no single reason why they should dull pain – or affect different parts of the body – but it is thought that it could be due partly to the anti-inflammatory, circulatory and detoxifying effects of some oils and the anaesthetic effect of others (Price & Price, 1999 p.68). Some essential oils have sedative or soporific (encourages sleep) effects which ease pain – bergamot, chamomile (Roman) and ylang ylang (Rossi *et al*, 1988). An analgesic effect may also be due to specific components, as for example, eugenol (a component in clove bud oil), which is well known to be effective on toothache.

Pain expresses itself in many of the emotions we experience, especially in grief, which is a complicated emotion, for which any essential oil with an analgesic action should be effective. When we are deeply angry at ourselves, or are suffering from the pain of guilt, it would be worth our while to use an essential oil with analgesic properties.

Analgesic Essential Oils

- aniseed
- black pepper
- coriander
- fennel
- geranium
- juniper
- marjoram (sweet)
- nutmeg
- pine
- sage

- basil
- clove bud
- eucalyptus (smithii)
- frankincense
- ginger
- lavender
- niaouli
- peppermint
- rosemary
- tea tree

Antifungal and Antiviral

Several investigations have been carried out on essential oils to discover which have fungicidal effects, and it was found in three separate research studies that aldehydes and esters were the two components that were especially effective in this field (Maruzella, 1961, Thompson & Cannon, 1986, Larrondo & Calvo, 1991). Some oils have general antifungal properties, whilst others affect specific fungi, such as, *Candida albicans* and *Tinea pedis* (athlete's foot).

Many essential oils have been tested for their effects on different viruses, and although several have been found to be efficient in this direction, no-one knows exactly which components are responsible. For example, 12 components from a wide range of oils were found to be active against both herpes simplex viruses, showing that there is no one component responsible.

I believe jealousy is like a fungus or a virus attacking us; something we don't really need or want, but comes to those of us who are vulnerable to desire – of things we cannot have, of someone else's partner or of a job someone else in the office secured that we really wanted (destructive and negative). On the other hand, it may be due to a desire for the same physical attributes as a friend, or indeed, those of their personality, like self-confidence (destructive, but not negative).

Because of this 'attack' on our better selves, I feel it is reasonable to expect that an oil which is effective on a physical fungus or virus could be effective on a mental fungus or virus also. Unfortunately, people who experience negative jealousy or envy (not quite the same thing, but similar) do not like to admit it to other people, so I have no first-hand experience of effectiveness on clients. If a reader has personal success with the oils I am suggesting, it would be in everyone's interests to let me know; I would not use your name, just as I have not used the real names of client cases appearing in this book – or in any other I have written.

Antifungal Essential Oils

- basil
- clove bud
- mandarin
- patchouli
- pine
- sage
- thyme (sweet)

- clary sage
- geranium
- lavender
- peppermint
- rosemary
- tea tree

Antiviral Essential Oils

- basil
- clove bud
- lavandin
- niaouli
- rosemary
- tea tree

- bergamot
- eucalyptus (smithii)
- lemon
- peppermint
- sage
- thyme (sweet)

Anti-inflammatory

Certain essential oils have been shown to have anti-inflammatory effects (Jackovlev *et al*, 1983) and numerous inflammatory conditions (conditions ending in 'itis') can be helped by oils containing this property. It is invaluable in cases of skin inflammations and arthritis, to say nothing of internal inflammation as in bronchitis, sinusitis and cystitis.

As anger is an inflamed condition of the mind, we would expect an anti-inflammatory essential oil to soothe anger and even the milder, linked conditions such as impatience and frustration.

Anti-inflammatory Essential Oils

- basil
- fennel
- geranium
- lavender
- melissa
- orange (bitter)
- peppermint
- pine
- rosemary
- thyme (sweet)

- chamomile (Roman and German)
- frankincense
- juniper
- lemon
- niaouli
- patchouli
- petitgrain
- rose otto (distilled)
- tea tree
- yarrow

Antispasmodic

Some essential oils, tested in 1964 by Debelmas & Rochat, were found to relieve cramp in smooth muscle fibres (those which are in the digestive tract) and further tests corroborated this (Debelmas & Rochat, 1967, Taddei *et al*, 1988). Over the years, I have had exceptional results on clients with skeletal muscle cramp using sweet marjoram and basil and two French friends of mine who have written a medical book on aromatherapy recommend cypress, which I have since tried and found to be successful (Franchomme & Pénoël, 1990).

I believe that essential oils with an antispasmodic action will release the tight, cramping feeling of anger, and as guilt could also make us feel cramped inside, the antispasmodic action would be appreciated here too. With fear, our muscles actually become physically tight – and although they may not be cramped as such, the antispasmodic action will help to relax the tight feeling – and accentuate any calming action the oil we have chosen may also have on the mind. We suffer emotional cramp if our mind dwells for too long on whatever is causing our fear, indicating that these same properties are needed to give us relief.

If any life experience which 'cramps our style' is making us unhappy, and you use essential oils regularly, try those which have antispasmodic properties!

Antispasmodic Essential Oils

- aniseed
- bergamot
- chamomile (Roman and German)
- coriander
- fennel
- geranium
- lemon
- mandarin
- nutmeg
- petitgrain
- sage
- ylang ylang
- basil
- cajeput
- clary sage
- clove bud
- cypress
- frankincense
- lavender
- marjoram (sweet)
- melissa
- peppermint
- rosemary
- thyme (sweet)

Anticatarrhal

In order to kill and get rid of the germs causing catarrh, essential oils containing powerful components called ketones, and sometimes lactones, are needed. These are capable of breaking down mucus so that we can expel it more easily. Certain oils, in research carried out in 1938 (Gordonoff), 1946 (Boyd & Pearson) and 1985 (Schilcher) were found to be effective as expectorants (the medical term for medicaments which help us to cough up mucus).

The association with the emotion of guilt is quite easy to understand, as is the association with anger, when you want to 'get it off your chest'. Essential oils with a releasing effect on catarrh are needed by people who are feeling guilty after loss of a loved one – 'did I do enough?', 'if only I had . . .' – and when anger is within, like this kind of guilt, we need to release it in order to heal ourselves.

Anticatarrhal Essential Oils

- aniseed
- cajeput
- fennel
- juniper
- melissa
- pine
- sandalwood
- thyme (sweet)
- basil
- cypress
- geranium
- lavender
- patchouli
- rosemary
- tea tree
- yarrow

Balancing

Essential oils have remarkable balancing powers, evident by the fact that several of them not only energize and/or stimulate, but also calm and/or sedate. This seems curious and perplexing, but research has confirmed this ability (Torii, 1988) and it is known as the adaptogenic effect (Price & Price, 1999 p.75). Later on we look at essential oils which are neurotonic and essential oils which are calming and sedative, when the individual attribute is needed. Here, we are looking at essential oils where *both* of these properties are in the one oil.

Grief is one of the emotions where a 'double action' oil is most helpful. As it is such a variable emotion and it encompasses other emotions within it, grief requires not only versatility but a balancing action as well.

Balancing essential oils are naturally ideal healers where emotional imbalance, mood swings or irrationality are prevalent. This extraordinary balancing power also comes into its own with secondary emotions such as confusion and its partners – bewilderment, indecisiveness and uncertainty – all of which are often experienced in the grieving process too.

Balancing Essential Oils (Relaxing and Stimulating)

- basil
- clary sage
- geranium
- bergamot
- cypress
- lavender

- marjoram
- rose otto
- petitgrain

Cardiotonic

There is not much research on cardiotonic properties any essential oils may have, although there is evidence and experience in France concerning this (Franchomme & Pénoël, 1990). In England, essential oils have been shown to slow down an accelerated heart beat and relieve palpitations (rapid and forceful contraction of the heart) (Woolfson & Hewitt, 1992). Essential oils which are general tonics must also include this effect on the heart – thus I have favoured such oils in my choice.

There are several primary emotions where using an essential oil which is a tonic to the heart – thereby strengthening it – would be beneficial. In grief, our spirits are naturally low, and in addition to essential oils which uplift the nervous system, those which will boost and refresh a sorrowful heart, giving us the stamina to carry on, would be emotionally profitable. For fear, especially dread, the heart is in need of a boost – and cardiotonic oils would certainly be of use here. Oils which are capable of slowing down a fast-beating heart would also be useful if the circumstances were such that a fast-beating heart was a symptom. Guilt makes the heart heavy, so again a tonic, giving a lightening effect, would indicate an essential oil with cardiotonic properties. Where fear and guilt are intertwined with grief, I would suggest finding an essential oil with cardiotonic properties and looking at its other properties to see if it is also a nerve tonic, thus enhancing the possibility of success.

Cardiotonic oils would also benefit secondary emotions such as apathy, confusion and timidity, where strength, stamina and courage are the required qualities.

Cardiotonic Essential Oils

- aniseed
- fennel
- rosemary
- thyme (sweet)
- basil
- lavender
- sandalwood

Cicatrizant

Cicatrizant means healing. One of the healing properties of lavender is for burns. Lavender has additional healing properties shared by several other essential oils, helping in the healing of damaged tissue, such as ulcers, wounds and scars. If the oils are used in application to the skin, an efficient carrier would be St John's wort (hypericum) as this macerated oil was much used in the past for the treatment of burns and wounds (Weiss, 1998).

A number of emotions have need of healing oils, an excellent example being the grieving process, where the wounds can take a long time to heal. The scars left by guilt also require healing, and when anger has been 'boiling' within for any length of time, the essential oils specializing in healing boils and ulcers would be appropriate. The self-inflicted wounds of jealousy would also benefit from a healing approach.

Cicatrizant Essential Oils

- bergamot
- chamomile (Roman and German)
- geranium
- lemon
- rose otto
- sage
- cedarwood
- clove bud
- frankincense
- lavender
- patchouli
- rosemary

Circulatory

A few essential oils are endowed with the power to increase the rate at which blood flows through our bodies. Having a good blood circulation keeps us healthy, as blood not only brings nourishment to every one of our cells, but also takes away waste matter and toxins (helped by the lymph – another circulating body fluid). If there is congestion in the body, the circulation will be poor and organs will not be receiving sufficient nourishment, nor having the waste matter removed before it starts affecting the body health-wise. Bad eating habits, lack of exercise and stress are all contributory factors in slowing down the circulation. Gradually, with the build up of 'trapped' toxins, our health deteriorates and if prolonged, disease can set in (Price, 1999).

Secondary emotions such as apathy and timidity would benefit from circulation-stimulating essential oils, to get them going – they need as many stimulating effects as they can get! The primary – and destructive – emotion of jealousy could also be helped by circulation-stimulant oils, to help rid the mind of 'toxic' thoughts.

Circulation-stimulant Essential Oils (Blood and Lymph)

- benzoin
- cedarwood
- geranium
- orange (bitter)
- sage
- black pepper
- cypress
- lemon
- rosemary

Decongestant

Individual essential oils relieve congestion in different systems of the body. Regarding the reproductive system essential oils are needed which will relieve congestion, painful and difficult menstruation (dysmenorrhoea); in the circulatory system certain essential oils decongest the venous circulation, making the return of blood to the heart easier and faster and therefore relieving varicose veins and other problems of congested blood, such as bruises. Some essential oils have decongestant properties which relieve headaches and migraines; others relieve the congestion of a sluggish digestion and yet others relieve catarrhal congestion in asthmatical and bronchial problems.

Several emotions present symptoms of congestion, when the mind is 'clogged' with too many thoughts to present a clear picture of what to do, as in some aspects of guilt and grief, when confusion may also be experienced. When the mind needs to be cleared, as in uncertainty, bewilderment or indecisiveness, decongestant oils can be very advantageous.

Decongestant Essential Oils

- cajeput
- chamomile (German)

- clary sage
- patchouli
- pine
- sandalwood

- geranium
- peppermint
- rosemary

Detoxifying, Purifying

When the body has a build-up of toxic matter, due to incorrect eating or drinking habits, lack of exercise and so on, several organs can suffer: the lymph, into which toxins are deposited for expulsion; the kidneys, which also receive toxins to be excreted; and the liver, our largest organ, which takes on toxins from alcohol over-consumption and residual toxic matter resulting from too many medicaments (as in my mother's case).

Emotions such as jealousy, revenge, greed and certain forms of guilt, such as a troubled conscience, which are mental toxins, would benefit from essential oils which can detoxify our physical body, cleansing us and giving us a new start.

Detoxifying Essential Oils

- clary sage
- juniper
- rosemary

Diuretic

There is evidence that one or two essential oils are diuretic, Gattefossé (1937 p.71) going as far as to say that nearly all essential oils are diuretic. Diuretic essential oils are effective on obesity, cellulite and oedema (infiltration of watery fluid into the tissues), typified when under the skin by soft, usually painless, swelling and often evident during pregnancy – more painful is the fluid swelling round the joints, as in rheumatism. Diuretic oils are also helpful in urinary disorders and where insufficient urine is being excreted, as can happen when certain medicaments are being taken for high blood pressure.

Wherever an emotion is being held inside and needs to be

released, diuretic oils would be beneficial. They would be indicated for all primary emotions which have been held deep inside or continually suppressed – grief, anger, fear and guilt and even jealousy, long held, could benefit from the use of diuretic essential oils.

Diuretic Essential Oils

- aniseed
- cypress
- lemon
- marjoram
- sage
- thyme (sweet)

- caraway
- fennel
- juniper
- rosemary
- sandalwood

Digestive

Several essential oils have strong effects on the digestive system – in different ways. Did you know that apéritif drinks contain essential oils to help stimulate both appetite (if necessary!) and digestive secretions, so that food is digested more easily and happily, because the oils selected usually possess antibacterial and antispasmodic properties too? Many apéritif-type oils are from a plant family whose essential oils are usually confined to professional use, though if used carefully, and only as recommended, there are no hazards.

Some digestive essential oils can relieve nausea and nervous vomiting and, also in the digestive category, come those oils which have been found to be effective on indigestion and flatulence (wind). There are far too many digestive system references for me to name them here, though they are in the book I wrote together with my husband on aromatherapy for health professionals.

The digestive system slows down when experiencing fear, in order to give extra energy to the rest of the body; it therefore makes sense, when fear has established itself, to stimulate the digestive system as a whole – to revitalize it. Oils which stimulate the appetite would be helpful during the grieving process, as food is often furthest from the mind – and I believe that any essential oils with stimulant powers would be helpful where apathy has taken hold of someone's life.

When the mind is experiencing guilt, it is often 'congested' with conflicting and often painful thoughts; this same type of congestion is also a symptom of deep fear. Oils which relieve painful indigestion should therefore be included in the final choice, to help relieve these emotions.

With flatulence, the body has air trapped in the digestive system, wanting to escape. Sometimes, with guilt feelings and those of hidden anger, we would like to 'get it out into the open'; what better to help this than carminative (gas-releasing) essential oils? With a complicated emotion like grief, other emotions can surface, and if there is any feeling that needs to be released, oils with this property may be needed *(see Chapter 7 for individual digestive effects)*.

Digestive Essential Oils

- basil
- black pepper
- coriander
- geranium
- juniper
- mandarin
- melissa
- niaouli
- orange (bitter)
- rosemary
- bergamot
- chamomile
- fennel
- ginger
- lemon
- marjoram
- neroli
- nutmeg
- peppermint
- sage

Hormone-like

There are several essential oils which, although not hormonal (that is, they are not comparable with the hormones in our body), have a tendency to normalize hormonal secretions when these are out of balance.

> There are compounds in some volatile essential oils which have structures similar to natural human hormones, and these promote efficient endocrine gland activity by natural means.
>
> Price & Price, p.79

Some oils have a balancing action on the reproductive system where they can benefit the ovaries, menstruation, breastfeeding, menopausal and sexual problems. Others are cortisone-like (Franchomme & Pénoël, p.87), some affect the adrenal glands and some the thyroid gland.

Hormonal imbalance is known to affect the emotions – as in PMS and the menopause – and in both of these women can suffer from mood swings, sometimes to the detriment of their relationship with their partner or/and children, as well as friends and acquaintances. Using essential oils to balance these states is therefore beneficial to everyone concerned.

Hormone-like Essential Oils

- aniseed
- chamomile (German)
- clove bud
- fennel
- niaouli
- pine
- sage

- cajuput
- clary sage
- cypress
- marjoram
- peppermint
- rosemary
- thyme (sweet)

Immunostimulant

The original cause of a depleted immune system is often a high stress level or deep depression. Immunostimulant essential oils can stimulate an immune system which is not functioning well. When depression is added to chronic illnesses like post-viral fatigue syndrome (ME), cancer and HIV, the need for such oil is greater.

Grief is probably the emotion most in need of immunostimulant essential oils; depression can so easily occur, and as many other emotions are involved, without intervention the resistance of the body would be lowered considerably, eventually threatening both physical and emotional health. Only the individuals concerned would be able to tell if their guilt was serious or long-standing enough to affect their resistance to ill-health. If such people found themselves continually succumbing to common colds or headaches, I would suggest using an immune-strengthening essential oil.

Immunostimulant Essential Oils

- clove bud
- lemon
- tea tree
- patchouli
- frankincense
- niaouli
- thyme (sweet)

Litholytic

This means the ability to break down stones – in the kidneys or in the gall bladder – and several essential oils have the ability to do this.

Forgiveness is not an emotion, but it is a means of releasing emotions like anger; it is often difficult to forgive people who have hurt us, but if we resist forgiveness we can become 'hard' inside. An unforgiving spirit – and possibly jealousy (which is a 'hard' emotion) – can be softened by the use of litholytic oils, making the lives of those concerned more pleasant in the case of forgiveness – and our own lives more pleasant in both cases.

Litholytic Essential Oils

- fennel
- lemon
- pine
- juniper
- niaouli
- rosemary

Mental Stimulant

Only a few oils are mentally stimulating and they are extremely useful in cases of lost memory or when we need help to remember facts – as in an examination, for example.

Mentally-stimulating essential oils are a great advantage in emotions such as all forms of grief and fear. Secondary emotions such as apathy, timidity and confusion can also benefit from mental stimulation.

Mental Stimulant Essential Oils

- clove
- peppermint
- rosemary

Neurotonic

It is fortunate that there is a fairly long list of essential oils which are neurotonic (tonic to the nerves). These oils are invaluable to help lift people out of depressive states, and if depression features strongly in any illness, the essential oils on which to base the final choice are those with this ability to uplift the spirits. Many neurotonic oils are multi-functional, benefiting not only general fatigue and debility, but also conditions such as insomnia, indigestion, nausea and hair loss when these are nervous in origin.

Their link with emotions is clear. For example, when fear first takes hold, we often get a 'sick feeling in the stomach'; it therefore makes sense, if we are in this situation, to use those neurotonic essential oils which have the ability to 'settle' or resolve this unpleasant experience.

Neurotonic oils are valuable for their beneficial effects on grief, which is always threatened with the development of depression; they are needed at all times to keep the spirits as high as is possible under the circumstances. Certain oils with this property can assist with insomnia when this is linked with the nerves, as is often the case in grief.

Neurotonic oils are useful for the many different forms which apathy can take *(see Chapter 7)* and they can be employed to strengthen people in the various manifestations of timidity.

Neurotonic Essential Oils

- basil
- clary sage
- coriander
- frankincense
- lavender
- bergamot
- clove bud
- cypress
- juniper
- marjoram

- neroli
- pine
- rosemary
- thyme (sweet)

- nutmeg
- rose otto
- sage

Relaxing, Sedative

Essential oils with these properties are a blessing in all cases of anxiety and stress, including many of the symptoms they portray, such as sleeplessness and headaches, nightmares, agitation, irritability and nervous shock. If anxiety or stress is behind the ailment showing itself, the essential oils on which to base the final choice are those which have a relaxing or calming action.

One of the main emotional experiences which has need of these oils is that of anger – and all the various forms it can take. Fear also needs calming oils when stress is the ruling feature; however, in states of terror and panic, the stronger calming oils – those which are also sedative – would be more efficient. In the grieving process, when everything seems 'just too much', calming essential oils are most effective – and when anger or fear are also experienced at this time, these oils are essential.

People who are given to daydreaming, or are continually with 'head in the clouds', require in particular the stronger, sedative essential oils; these are more effective in bringing them down to earth – or 'grounding' them, as the expression is in some complementary therapies.

Relaxing, Sedative Essential Oils

- aniseed
- bergamot
- chamomile (Roman)
- geranium
- lavender
- mandarin
- neroli
- petitgrain
- ylang ylang

- basil
- caraway
- cypress
- juniper
- lemon
- melissa
- orange (bitter)
- sandalwood

Conclusion

This chapter has shown how the application of holism in the practical sense can bring about the relief of emotional difficulties by careful and studied choice to find the relevant essential oils. If you ask yourself appropriate questions regarding your physical and mental aspects, to reveal your true state, then it is possible to arrive at a selection of healing essential oils which will improve your overall health – in mind, body and spirit.

6 States of Mind which Affect the Emotions

Sing praise to the Lord,
  all his faithful people!
Remember what the Holy One has done,
  and give him thanks!
His anger lasts only a moment,
  his goodness for a lifetime.
Tears may flow in the night,
  but joy comes in the morning.

Psalm 30: 4/5

According to psychologists, the life of an emotion is very short –
often only a few seconds; at most, several minutes. Emotions which
last longer than a few minutes could actually be a number of different individual sets of responses which happen over and over again
(Lindenfield, 1997 p.21). One thing is evident: emotions are very
complex. For example, whilst experiencing jealousy, it is possible also
to experience shame, anger and hatred – and more, which, if the psychologists are right, would change and alternate with each other all
the time.

One particular emotion has to 'start us off' and is an automatic
response from the brain to the 'feeling' part of the mind. Usually the
brain triggers an immediate action by the body, such as:

a) running away from something which has frightened us;
*as a child – and even as a young adult – Susan was frightened of drunk-
en men; if she saw one as far as 30 feet away, she would panic and rush
to the other side of the street to avoid passing him.*

By running away, which was the action triggered by the brain on experiencing her fear, Susan had avoided further anxiety, though she had not solved her emotional problem.

b) welcoming something which delights us;
Marion was missing her husband, who was away on business for two weeks. After 10 days, she received a phone call from his firm to say he would be home in a few hours. Filled with joy, she dashed out to buy his favourite wine and made his favourite dish, to show her pleasure.

The telephone call had lifted Marion's sadness to joy and expectation, giving her the energy to act – and prepare everything in the short time available to her.

c) resolving something which has confused us;
Pauline was giving a lecture and had been given all the details; where, when and for how long. A week before the lecture she received a letter which contradicted some of the parameters she had been given originally. She was confused and panicked a little; her action was to telephone her contact number to resolve the situation.

Pauline experienced relief after the telephone call (which was the action initiated by her anxiety); her emotional experience was fleeting, unlike Susan's emotional obsession, which needed help to make it disappear from the back of her mind.

It is not as easy to select essential oils for emotional problems as it is to select them for physical health disorders – and, of course, in cases like Marion's, there is no need of them, though she could have vaporized a mix of essential oils to relax and give them both extra pleasure.

Most research done on essential oils in the past has been on their bactericidal and antiseptic properties, although more recently, studies have been carried out to prove their effectiveness on health disorders such as insomnia, rheumatism and stress. Apart from research which shows that essential oils do have an effect on the mind (relaxing or stimulating), there is no substantiated evidence for their effects on individual emotions. Thus, the choice in books on this subject has depended on the personal experience of writers who are practitioners of aromatherapy – and, of course, anyone else in practice who has reported their results.

At every single place where I lecture (and there are many – both in the UK and abroad) I make a plea to the therapist audiences for case studies to print in *The Aromatherapist* or *Aromatherapy World* (journals for therapists) as these are the only 'evidence' we can have at the moment in the absence of clinical tests. I ask for them not for myself, but in the interests of all aromatherapists, as by reading of someone else's experience, the readers themselves may be able to help one of their own clients. However, I am sorry to say that these impassioned pleas rarely receive a response – yes! I do get some case studies, but these are usually sent in to the Shirley Price International College of Aromatherapy as part of an advanced diploma – in other words, because they *had* to do it! It is only a very small proportion of what *could* be available as a record of single case studies in the interest of aromatherapy and to provide a reason for someone to do a clinical trial.

Do not forget that to get the best results from the essential oils you have chosen *(see Chapters 5, 6 and 7)*, you should look at your whole lifestyle, otherwise it is a bit like driving a car with the hand-brake on; it still goes, but not at full potential. Check the following, and if any apply to you, do something about them *at the same time* as using the oils of your choice, so that you can benefit at full potential:

- eat wisely, give up smoking if you can, take alcohol and coffee in moderation – otherwise in the long-term you only make matters worse
- take regular exercise – even if it is only half an hour a day. You can vary it if you don't like routine. Take a walk around the block, clean a window (very good exercise – and slimming!), go swimming, wash the kitchen floor. There are many things you can do for exercise so try to make it something that you enjoy
- know how to stop when you're tired; no one performs well when they are tired – and pushing yourself will only increase the stress. This is the time to relax a little; do some breathing exercises and read a book or watch TV (not a horror movie!)
- have a warm bath with relaxing essential oils and a warm drink before going to bed
- make a list of things you have to do in order of their importance – and do one thing at a time with your full concentration

- delegate whatever you can that will not cause you extra worry
- be realistic about perfection; there is no need to be slipshod, but accept that a third or fourth draft of a letter which was due yesterday is only giving you extra stress; in the end, the last draft may not even be as good as the first.

Stress and Depression

Before looking at the individual emotions which affect us adversely, and arranging them in groups, we need to consider the main states of mind which can alter or initiate emotions, or indeed, be altered by them – stress and depression. These seem to be omnipresent in our modern society – not that they are new experiences, but people nowadays are more aware of them. Although the following quote refers only to depression, it could as easily be true about stress as well – the italics are mine:

> I must emphasise that *stress*, depression and hopelessness are not emotions per se; they can be chronic mental states that result from our inability to integrate emotions. Once we acknowledge, express and resolve feelings such as sadness and anger, we are generally less likely to become *stressed*, depressed or hopeless.
>
> Domar & Dreher 1997

Stress and depression are relative terms describing how an individual is 'feeling' compared to his or her ordinary experience of life. As we are all individuals, the feelings one person would describe as ordinary may be debilitating to somebody else. This can mean that those around a person suffering from depression or stress may be intolerant of that person; they cannot appreciate how the circumstances are oppressive to that particular individual because the same set of circumstances would not have affected them in the same way. It is easy to look into a person's situation when the experiences are not our own, and think we know what they should do, or decide on how they should deal with aspects of their lives which are causing them anxiety.

When stress is chronic, it can be a cause of depression. Many depressive and highly stressful states are brought about by a severe life event (like the death of a loved one) or a major difficulty (like living with a drunken husband) – in other words, a provoking factor. Whether or not this turns to depression depends on the vulnerability of the person concerned and the number of difficulties arising at any one time, for instance, losing one's mother at the same time as going through a divorce at the same time as having three young children to care for on one's own. Price (1994) discovered that the effects of multiple stress often resulted in thinning hair or hair loss, which naturally increased the depressive state. Brown & Harris (1978) bear this theory out with their story of a woman with three teenage children living at home and having the following composite problems to cope with, causing both stress and depression to set in:

• she was a widow
• there was no heating or lighting in the house because she couldn't afford to pay for the electricity and gas
• her 16-year-old son was on probation for violence and, as if this was not a severe enough life event to have to suffer all at one time, without a husband's support
• she was told that she would be put in jail if she couldn't pay the 16-year-old's fine of £400. She was completely without hope.

In severe cases of stress and/or depression, mental exhaustion or fatigue can set in. The underlying anxiety and all the accompanying states of mind can be treated effectively with essential oils – with or without massage. However, as each essential oil is capable of a variety of health effects, both mental and physical, there is quite a long list of essential oils which could be beneficial, therefore the final choice depends on:

• which emotions are being experienced most of the time
• whether or not any physical symptoms are also presenting themselves.

Aromatherapy is particularly beneficial to both stress and depression, as one of its main aims is to bring balance and harmony to the mind. Essential oils are balancing substances (especially those containing esters, *see Chapter 5)* and, as such, help the *whole* person to adjust to his/her particular situation in life:

In the tradition of aromatherapy, specific essential oils are stress reducing, whereas others are energising, and still others can have either effect, depending on the user's state of mind/body interaction ... We reasoned the best way for us to study the stress-reducing properties of fragrance would be to investigate their physiological effects.

Warren & Warrenburg, 1993

If stress or depression (or both, as they are often interrelated) are responsible for how you are feeling, you should first write down all the oils which are listed below for your state of mind. If you are also extremely tired all the time or suffering from mental exhaustion, put a tick against the oils which will help these conditions too – if they are not already on your list, add them to it.

This is the basis on which the final choice will be made. The next step is to see if any of those oils will also help alleviate any other emotional or physical problem you may have; if they will, tick these too. Always select more than one oil, for synergy (see Chapter 9), and if there are too many to choose from, select those whose aroma is most pleasing to you, as this is an important consideration.

Sometimes action is needed for sudden emotions like panic or shock as a result of upsetting news. Neroli and rose otto are the ones usually recommended for this. For hysteria, melissa and rosemary have been cited (Price & Price, 1999).

CASE STORY

Margaret's mother, who is a chronic asthmatic, had a sudden and serious attack while washing up one night on their boat. She panicked, as she had left her inhaler (which she used in emergencies) at home. Fortunately, Margaret had her mother's asthma mix of essential oils in her handbag. She always carried neroli with her because she loved it so much, and while she rubbed the asthma mix onto her mother's upper back and appropriate feet reflexes, she gave her mother the neroli to inhale deeply. This immediately reduced her panic somewhat, and the essential oils kept her breathing from getting any worse until they reached the shore (next to the house), where Margaret's sister ran to fetch the inhaler.

Anxiety and Worry

Anxiety (a state of apprehension) and worry (an over-anxious state of mind) are often the forerunners of both stressful and depressive states – in fact, the body has the same initial reaction as in the first stage of stress *(see below)*. A mild form of stress (now a medical condition), anxiety and worry can take two forms:

a) reaction to a potentially harmful situation; it is perfectly natural and healthy to experience anxiety when faced with danger or risk of some kind. Together with fear, it enables the body to deal with the situation by increasing the respiratory and heart rate, thus extra oxygen reaches the brain; it also releases energy and extra adrenalin, to help cope with the situation. For example:
you see your child fall from the branch of a tree. Your extra adrenalin and energy enable you to dash out of the house (heart pounding) to see how seriously he is hurt. You are worried that he may have broken a bone, so you take him to hospital. Your anxiety is relieved immediately when the doctor tells you he is not seriously hurt.

b) reaction to an ongoing life event; here the anxious feeling or worry may be connected to work, a problematic marriage, illness, a son in the army who is sent into battle, etc. This sort of anxiety, if the situation becomes serious, usually develops into either stress or (and) depression, depending on the personality of the person.

Essential Oil Choice

For all forms of anxiety, essential oils which will relax both mind and body are the obvious choice *(see oils for 'Stress', below)*. If the anxiety contains within it an element of fear, the essential oils reputed to help dispel fear must also be considered; look at fear (page 138) and see if any of the relaxing oils also contain properties which will help allay fear. In an ongoing situation, the mind is often overactive, therefore the choice should include those oils which could reduce 'production' so to speak, such as oils with astringent or styptic properties *(See Chapter 5)*.

If you know you are the 'worrying kind' then you should use

essential oils at the first signs of anxiety to keep you calm *now* – and help prevent the situation developing into stress.

Stress

Stress has been called 'the disease of the 80s' (Topping, 1990) – but what exactly is it? You may feel stressed at this very moment, as you are reading these words! There may be things which have happened today that have caused you tension or anxiety; problems concerning money, family or work (or the lack of it); things which you yourself cannot control or influence may have added to your stress, such as the battery failing in your alarm clock, causing you to miss an important 'first of the day' appointment.

According to the Canadian physician Hans Selye (1984) and other experts on stress, prolonged stress provokes first an immediate reaction, then a more or less balanced state in which the stress is resisted – and finally there is a breakdown of this resistance (Wingate & Wingate, 1988), when health begins to be affected.

Positive and Negative Stress

Stress is not always negative or even unwelcome; indeed, a certain amount of stress is necessary in order for us to function efficiently and can be coped with; a certain amount is positive and may even be wanted. Stress is only negative when it is unwanted or excessive. In the first instance the body uses stress as a motivator and as a coping mechanism. In fact, there may be more than a little truth in the saying 'don't ask me to relax – it's my stress that keeps me together!'.

The production of adrenalin is one of the positive side-effects of stress which we need – to motivate us and give us energy to do even the simplest of tasks. Stress is therefore not necessarily a problem – it only becomes so when we have more stress than we can cope with in the normal run of life. Its depth is reflected by the rate of wear and tear in the body caused by life (Selye, 1984). In other words, it is a dependent experience – dependent on the measure of life's suffering, or enjoyment. Stress, like the emotions, can be labelled productive and unproductive, or positive and negative. A sportsperson experiences pleasurable, positive stress during a competitive game or when climbing Mount Everest. Positive stress stimulates us, giving us the energy to cope with challenging or demanding tasks like these, after which both body and mind return to their normal composure without having had any negative effect on our health.

On the other hand, negative stress can cause frustration and irritability to take hold – even moodiness – and if not taken in hand, can weaken our resistance to ill-health. Some people may go through life suffering only mild stresses, with which they can cope, having only minor disorders which do not seriously affect their health. Others may suffer such severe stress that they become ill, either physically, mentally – or both – depending on the 'rate of wear and tear' the particular stress exerts on their bodies or minds.

It is possible, in one sense, to compare stress with the common cold. How many people, when they have a bad cold, say they have flu – and how many do you know who say they are 'really stressed' when in reality they are just a bit 'pushed'? As I said above, without a certain amount of stress, none of us could function to our best ability.

How Does the Body Deal with Stress?

The body deals with all stress (both positive and negative) by releasing extra energy from our nutritional 'store'. At the same time, extra oxygen is transported to the brain and extra adrenalin produced. These changes within our bodies prepare us to cope with a situation causing immediate stress. This preparation is what Hans Selye calls the first stage of stress. The second stage is the action we take using these extra resources. For example:

A mother has lost her small child whilst shopping; she cannot see him but is not too worried as she searches in the aisle she is in. He is not there – and stress (stage one) commences. She runs down every aisle, using the extra energy. Panic is now the emotion experienced by the child's mother – and the stress increases. If the child still cannot be found, fear is added to panic, which increases the stress. This will continue if neither the mother nor the store detective can find the child – on or off the premises. They telephone the police, and the stress becomes even more intense as another emotion – guilt (or self-blame) – may be experienced: 'why did I not keep hold of his hand'?

It is only when a stressful situation is prolonged – and is not treated at this stage – that the third stage, starting with exhaustion, commences. As this is a hypothetical story, we can give it a happy ending; someone had found the child wandering in the street outside and had taken him to the police station. The intense emotion of relief may have caused yet another emotion – anger – to be experienced by the mother; how many of us have been 'angry' with our child just because we are relieved that they have emerged from a situation which has worried us? Nevertheless, this stressful situation was fortunately terminated, so the mother's body and mind would gradually return to normal.

Had the story above concerned a teenager missing after school, then not only the next day too, but perhaps for several weeks or months, a magnitude of emotions would be experienced and severe stress would set in. When excess of stress builds up like this, stage three commences – and true (clinical) stress is experienced. This can occur because of an emotional disturbance like the above, severe physical injury, illness or work overload – even a lack of any challenge in life – and manifests itself in headaches, stomach disorders, insomnia, susceptibility to infections, etc. due to the gradual closing down of the immune system (Price & Price, 1999 p.208).

How Should We Deal with Stress?

A common reaction to stress is to drink more coffee or smoke more cigarettes (if you are a smoker). This, unfortunately, does nothing to diminish the stress itself; it is much better to get to grips with it yourself, in a positive way. Plan your day carefully, so that there is time for a break; perhaps even a short walk, which in itself is relaxing. If a walk is not possible during the day, get up half an hour earlier (going to bed half an hour earlier if you need the sleep) and take a short walk before breakfast (this should be more than just a drink of tea or coffee, which is not a good start to the day, even for an unstressed person!). Take your time when eating – don't rush your food; this stresses your digestive system, so you are not doing yourself any favours.

Essential Oil Choice

Many essential oils contain natural chemical components which are relaxing, calming or sedative; it is from these that the initial choice should be made in order to tackle stress successfully.

> We reasoned the best way for us to study the stress-reducing properties of fragrance would be to investigate their physiological effects.
>
> Warren & Warrenburg, 1993

Oils which contain these necessary constituents (and which are among those detailed in Chapter 8) are:

- aniseed
- chamomile (Roman)
- clove bud
- juniper berry
- lemon
- melissa
- orange (bitter)
- ylang ylang
- bergamot
- clary
- cypress
- lavender
- marjoram (sweet)
- neroli
- rose otto

CASE STORY

Colin had recently changed his job to one which was not only more financially rewarding than his previous one, but which also enabled him to get out of the office and meet people. His reason for consulting me was to see if I could 'cure' the stye on his right eye, which he could get rid of with medication, but kept reappearing. Its frequent recurrence was frustrating him, especially as he was meeting people every day and wanted to look his best. His frustration was often expressed by irritation with his family, occasionally creating problems between him and his wife.

Through careful questioning about his job, I discovered that he had recently been nominated top salesman of the year – after only 11 months with the company. Winning this award entailed addressing his colleagues at sales meetings every so often throughout the year and the whole idea had filled him with apprehension. The stye had first made its appearance before the second weekly meeting (though he had not been asked to speak at either of these), and had been at its worst after the first time he had had to address his colleagues. A special meeting was to be held the week after his visit to me, at which he had been asked to speak, and he felt particularly anxious about this one; his eye had flared up again and on top of this he was not sleeping very well. Seeing that the stye, the irritation and the insomnia were stress based, I persuaded him to come for an aromatherapy treatment two days before his talk, giving him our Chamomile Eye Care to use three or four times a day until then. He returned for his appointment, rather nervous, as he had never before had a massage. He confessed that he had only come because the eye drops had already begun to clear his stye, which gave him the confidence to try at least a back massage.

The oils selected were three which would help his emotional symptoms, and at the same time help his insomnia. From the oils which relieve stress, the following were selected for the extra properties Colin needed:

- *Roman chamomile*, which would alleviate his frustration and irritation at home (analgesic and anti-inflammatory) and help him to sleep (calming)
- *lavender*, with the same properties as above
- *sweet marjoram*, which would aid his insomnia (calming) and ease his frustration and irritation (analgesic).

He telephoned three weeks later to make another appointment (for two days before his next lecture) because his stye had almost disappeared before his talk and had not reappeared (he was still using the drops daily). He also admitted to having felt reasonably relaxed while giving the talk!

At his third treatment, I discovered that his wife had remarked on his happier frame of mind. His improvement was such that I felt he could manage without further treatment, but should use the same essential oils in his bath and inhale them from a tissue the last four days before a talk, taking a tissue to inhale from just before giving each one. He returned for more oils sooner than expected, because his wife loved the aroma and was using them in her daily bath!

Depression

Depression seems to affect women more than men. Like stress, it is a much abused word, many people saying they are depressed, when in reality they are simply feeling temporarily sad, or low spirited; perhaps dejection or despondency would be more appropriate terms for this kind of 'depression'. Fortunately, after a relatively short period of, at most, several days, most of us 'snap out' of a temporary dejected state and are able to resume our normal 'emotional' lives.

When feeling low, emotional experiences change, and the longer the situation causing the despondency lasts, the more the likelihood of it developing into a true state of depression.

Depression takes in a whole range of melancholic dispositions, not least those connected with moodiness and apathy, as sufferers can feel lethargic, bored, suffer mood swings and often show little interest in anything at all. Other emotions can also play a part in the whole depressed state, such as sadness, grief, remorse and shame. Rita Carter (1998) says that depression is more than just a mood; because the brains of people who are depressed are less active than normal, it probably accounts for physical symptoms like fatigue and lethargy.

> There can be pain and disturbance of sleep and appetite, the memory is affected and thinking is slowed. Anxiety, irrational fear and agitation may be present and a depressed person typically feels guilty, worthless and unloved. Life seems pointless and the 'meaning' is missing from things.
>
> Carter, 1998

Before a person can be 'officially' diagnosed as depressed, two factors have to be confirmed:

- that the social life of the person is interfered with
- that the condition has been going on for at least two weeks – some clinicians say a month.

The symptoms a clinician looks for are:

- lack of energy – a feeling of being 'washed out' all the time
- sleep problems; difficulty in getting to sleep or waking early and unable to get back to sleep
- slowing down in everything they do
- irritation and inability to concentrate on things (Wood, 1990 p.64).

When depression becomes chronic, people feel that their situation is going to continue interminably; they feel helpless to do anything about it and can become mentally exhausted, as well as often being pessimistic, frequently withdrawing into themselves (Wood, 1990 pp.63–5).

One cause of depression can be lack of sunshine in winter. Incidentally, this is responsible for many suicidal feelings in Finland, for example, where daylight is progressively reduced after the autumn until there is complete darkness for a few months. The sun slowly reappears as spring approaches; and in summer there is no dark night and the flowers are open all the time. It must be quite an adjustment to make emotionally each year. Other causes can be a feeling of inadequacy, or inability to cope, as in post-natal depression; rejection, at work – perhaps in a new job – or in a sports club or drama group, where previously recognized talents are ignored or belittled; in fact, any worrying life event can cause us to feel dejected and, eventually, depressed.

Once depressed, research shows that people think in a negative way about themselves; they remember their mistakes more easily than their successes and unhappy memories more easily than happy ones (Martin & Clark, 1985).

The main cause of depression is illness, which can bring about different emotional experiences, even if the illness is a minor one; frustration at missing an important social function, or not being able to finish that urgent job at work. If the illness is chronic or hopeless, as well as a deeper and stronger frustration (perhaps due to immobility of various joints and muscles as in arthritis), fear, despair and possibly anger can be experienced.

Even minor illnesses like coughs and colds or general aches and pains can trigger feelings of despondency which can lead to depression. If someone does not make a full recovery after a viral illness like flu, for example, they are left feeling drained and without energy, which can change despondency into full-blown depression, called post-viral fatigue syndrome. ME (myalgic encephalomyelitis) is one such illness, though where this is not due to the retention of a virus, it is called chronic fatigue syndrome. Many more people suffer with this than with what Clive Wood calls 'pure' ME (Wood, 1990 p.70).

We have already discovered that an aromatherapist does not select essential oils on the basis of the symptoms being portrayed (unlike allopathic medicine), but first asks about past health history and lifestyle, finding out whether or not stress or depression are evident in any part of the person's life. S/he has also to be a good listener – a skill not many of us have, though it is needed whenever someone needs help, physical or emotional:

> Yes, listening is a form of communication that can be *heard* by the one whose heart needs to be comforted. We're not always able to offer people solutions to their problems, but just to listen to them can give them hope. Most of all, it is a way of loving others.
>
> Yoder, 1999

> When we hold our tongues and listen
> We communicate our care;
> For an open ear speaks volumes
> To a heart that's in despair.
>
> Sper

Depression is relative to life and in order to help anyone, it is necessary to be able to hear the clues.

Selecting Essential Oils

Essential oils which can relieve depression and stimulate the mind, because they are neurotonic and energizing, are:

- *aniseed*
- *bergamot*
- basil
- *chamomile (Roman)*

- *clary sage*
- frankincense
- juniper
- *marjoram (sweet)*
- *orange (bitter)*
- petitgrain
- rosemary
- sage
- thyme (sweet)

- *cypress*
- ginger
- *lavender*
- *neroli*
- peppermint
- pine
- *rose otto*
- sandalwood

You have probably noticed that many of the essential oils which help depression are the same as those which can relieve stress (I have put these in italics). This is because many oils have a balancing effect due to their ester content *(see Chapter 5)*. Another impressive point about essential oils is that each has many properties; those needed to lift someone out of a depressive state can target not only the depression (thus achieving the purpose for which you selected them), but also maintain equilibrium – and (if selected carefully and knowledgeably), help to heal any other physical or mental problem for which each has an affinity.

CASE STORY

Harry had been feeling a bit low for several months and was having one or two problems with his health – nothing too serious, just the occasional headache and stomach problem. He wasn't too keen on seeing the doctor 'for nothing' as he put it, so his wife suggested he went to see her aromatherapist (it took some persuasion, but in the end he agreed). As a result of her assessment and listening skills, Sheila (the aromatherapist, a previous student of ours) discovered that:

- Harry was quiet and rather shy, although his position at work suggested he was intelligent
- he was unsettled at work; his new manager frequently asked his advice, which entailed extra work. This was sometimes stressful, but his manager never acknowledged or gave him credit for it, indeed, often taking the credit himself

- Harry's colleague, in a similar position to Harry, with a much shorter length of service and never asked by the manager for advice of any kind, but popular, confident and always cracking jokes, was recently given the promotion Harry thought he would have had on account of having been so helpful over the last year
- his wife knew the situation and wanted him to find another job, but unfortunately his age was against him
- his physical symptoms were stomach cramps, sleeplessness and migraines, things he had never suffered from before the new manager had joined the company
- Sheila knew that he was sometimes irritable with his wife, as she had mentioned this to Sheila at her last treatment.

Because of his depressive state, Sheila looked at her list of antidepressant and uplifting oils. From these she selected three oils which would also help his physical symptoms. She selected, from the neurotonic oils:

- *basil,* which would alleviate his migraine (analgesic and antispasmodic) as well as helping his nervous insomnia (nervous system regulator); in addition its antispasmodic properties would relax his stomach cramps – an excellent choice for Harry
- *sweet marjoram,* which would relieve his migraines (analgesic and antispasmodic) and his insomnia (calming). Like basil, its antispasmodic properties would relax his digestive cramps – again, an excellent choice
- *frankincense,* an immunostimulant which is both energizing and strengthening to the nervous system.

Harry came to see her every two weeks, using the same oils at home in a vaporizer every night, a bath twice a week and on a tissue to inhale at work. Before he returned for his second treatment he was sleeping much better; on his third visit, he said he had realized that he hadn't had indigestion for over a week. When asked how he was coping at work, he said 'Well, I've just accepted the situation, but I feel stronger in myself – and actually told Geoff yesterday to give the piece of extra work he had asked me to do to my colleague – and he did!'
Harry's wife told Sheila she was absolutely delighted in the change

in her husband's attitude of mind – he had returned to his usual tolerant self, not once becoming touchy since his second treatment.

So, let us see now how Sheila's choice of oils was able to help Harry's emotional problems as well as his physical ones:

- all three oils are neurotonic and antidepressive
  they lifted his spirits, helping him to feel in a happier frame of mind
- all three oils are analgesic
  they relieved the hurt of not being chosen for promotion
- basil and marjoram are antispasmodic
  they worked on his irritability and also any unexpressed anger he may have experienced, but not told Sheila about
- marjoram is relaxing and calming
  it relieved the stress of the situation, helping him to accept it
- frankincense, with its energizing and mind strengthening properties, gave him the strength to cope with his manager's demands in a positive way.

Grouping Emotions

I have already said in Chapter 1 that defining emotions is not an easy task; some emotions could almost be defined as 'states of mind' and states of mind can produce (or perhaps *be*) emotions; they are very close. For instance, futility, hope, joy, escapism, gratitude, ingratitude, panic, loneliness, powerlessness, embarrassment, hostility, worry – all these are states of mind, like stress and depression, yet so strongly linked to the emotions that they could possibly even be described *as* emotions by some people. It becomes even more difficult when we talk about apathy and lethargy, which are often classed as emotions, yet as they continue for some considerable time, could as easily be described as states of mind.

As we know, every person is an individual, with different feelings and reactions to (and different coping abilities for) the same situation. It would be possible to put into groups people who have similar personalities, so that you can have a general, overall picture of the reaction of each group to a certain situation. To help you to understand how to select essential oils for your emotions, I am going to try and class the emotions together in the same sort of way, putting together those which seem to demonstrate similar basic sensitivities. This will give you (I hope!) a clearer concept of the overall picture and eliminate relying only on a long alphabetical list of seemingly unrelated emotions to find out which essential oils to use.

The following grouping is how I see it myself and is simply my opinion, not researched facts; it also represents feelings which are not easily separated from states of mind:

Basic Destructive States of Mind/Emotions

anxiety, apprehension, concern, consternation, distress, nervousness, tension, trepidation, uneasiness, worry

depression, deflation, dejection, despair, despondency, downheartedness, hopelessness, melancholy, sadness

stress, anxiety, pressure, strain, tension, trauma, worry

It is easy to see the link between feelings connected with anxiety and those connected with stress; now look at grief below and see how many of the emotions connected with grief are also experienced in depression.

Primary Emotions

grief, loss, sorrow, despair, hopelessness, hurt, despondency, disappointment

fear, lack of confidence, inferiority

anger, impatience, touchiness, irritability, frustration, annoyance, argumentativeness, negativity

jealousy, envy, revenge, suspicion, hatred, obsession, cynicism, blame

guilt, remorse, regret, shame

Secondary Emotions

moodiness, irrationality, emotional imbalance, brooding

apathy, lack of interest, boredom, lethargy

airy-fairy, not grounded, daydreaming, romantic

confusion, bewilderment, sense of loss – not belonging

timidity, sensitivity, shyness, cowardice, inadequacy, unworthiness, underachievement

Conclusion

When we can accept and resolve emotions which are destroying or diminishing ourselves and sometimes others, we are less likely to become stressed or depressed. This process is not always easy, and indeed, can be very difficult. By treating emotions before they become chronic, and looking seriously at our lifestyle, some pressures (which can lead to stress) and despondencies (which can lead to depression) can be avoided.

We need, if we can, to *choose* the state of mind we want to be in; unfortunately, some people never move on from a trauma because the trauma itself gives them purpose and identity and some kind of importance. Others, usually those with a positive frame of mind *(see Chapter 7)*, can move on without difficulty, because they are determined to. Using essential oils has been shown to help relax or stimulate the mind, and the case stories in this chapter (where essential oils have been used) demonstrate their efficacy in this respect.

7 *The Gamut of Emotions –*
Selecting Essential Oils for
Emotional Groups

Emotions can be further grouped into those which have characteristics in common with one another. Those appearing with the principal emotion in a particular group do not always denote exactly the same feeling, but are close enough as far as essential oil choice is concerned. Grouping emotions in this way is a great help when selecting essential oils, as it is less confusing and overwhelming than talking about each one separately.

Grief

> Even in laughter the heart may ache,
> and joy may end in grief.
>
> Proverbs 14:13

Grief, Despair, Disappointment, Hurt, Sense of Loss, Sorrow

- grief
  distress, deep sorrow, hurt, anguish, dejection
- despair
  to be without hope, anguish, wretchedness
- disappointment
  defeat of one's hopes or expectations, sadness
- hurt
  pain, wounded (by a remark), suffering, upset, sadness
- sense of loss
  deprivation, hurt
- sorrow
  anguish, distress, grief, sadness, dejection

See how grief, despair and sorrow all have anguish as an integral part of their suffering, and disappointment, hurt and distress all encompass sadness.

Grief, as I said in Chapter 1, is in itself a complex emotion. Perhaps this is why it is not often listed in a book on the mind or emotions, and is limited to articles or books on bereavement. It is a strong feeling, about which much can be written – perhaps grief is more a state of mind than an emotion? So much depends on the situation responsible for causing grief – and one's interpretation of the word.

> The most characteristic features of grief are the 'pangs' of severe anxiety and psychological pain which often end in outbursts of sobbing and crying. This should be looked upon as a release; it is far better to cry than to bottle up your grief by 'being brave'. Pangs of grief usually begin a few hours (sometimes days) after the bereavement and are at their peak between five and fourteen days.
>
> Murray-Parkes, 1986

Grief is an emotion which sooner or later needs to be expressed and resolved. Some relief can be brought by open, *relaxed* crying or talking about your grief to a close friend; without these two releasing actions, the full weight of the grief (and its adherent emotions which may apply) take much, much longer to dissipate. Domar and Dreher (1997 p.159) say that 'you won't free yourself from these manifestations until you confront grief directly'. Not an easy thing to do, but essential oils can be of great help in all aspects of grief.

CASE STORY

A friend of mine who is an aromatherapist and teacher of aromatherapy lost her baby granddaughter five years ago – her mother six months later. She bottled up her grief and used her work to 'get over it', working very hard indeed, filling her life with other things. During the following years, her health suffered seriously (including cancer and the necessary chemo- and radiotherapy treatments), though Brenda has worked through everything with the help of essential oils, her faith and positive thinking. Eventually, after a seriously bad back problem, she had to retire.

After a short while, she began to feel dejected and morose, so her husband took her away for a holiday to cheer her up. Brett had just completed the second part of his aromatherapy course, and to help Brenda's back, and her spirits, he gave her a massage every single day with essential oils of frankincense, Shirley lavender (as Brenda calls ours – her favourite lavender), rosemary and sandalwood (because she loves the aroma). A few days later, before they returned home, she found herself crying profoundly and realized she was at last expressing her grief.

That afternoon, she saw a baby deer, twice, on its own, without its mother, and the second time, the thought flashed through her head: 'if that baby deer knows where it's going without its mother and I don't, it's time I did something about it!' Since then, with the continued use of essential oils, her health – and spirits – have improved beyond recognition. In fact, when I saw her at our Open Day, I could hardly believe how well she looked and how bright and cheerful she was.

Let's look at some of the emotions which can surface at a time of grief caused by bereavement:

- shock
  whether or not the death was sudden – even expected – death is a shock
- deep sorrow and distress
  especially by those close to the bereaved
- anguish
  deep sense of loss, mental pain, loneliness – by a wife or husband, partner, son or daughter, very close friend
- remorse, regret
  of something which cannot now be put right; this is one of the worst emotions to feel after losing someone close and is almost impossible to come to terms with (Stephen, 1998)
- guilt
  perhaps there was more you could have done or said; a promise delayed and therefore unfulfilled

- anger
  yes – it's possible! 'How could he leave me with all these debts?'
  Or 'if only. . . ' directed at the nearest possible target – doctor,
  nurse, relative, employer, self. Sometimes it is the relatives who
  direct their anger – to the doctor, to the surviving loved one
- frustration
  'why didn't I . . . ?', 'I could have . . . '
- fear
  of being alone; of what people will say because he had just been
  put into a home
- confusion, bewilderment
  what happened? Why? Why him? What am I going to do?

It is important to the future well-being of the bereaved to try and
release emotions like regret, frustration, anger and guilt. Nothing you
think or worry about will bring about the resolution of the undone
things, so use positivity as well as essential oils to help release them.
It is not easy, but the grieving process takes an average of two years,
and if you can heal yourself of these destructive emotions, you will
adjust to your new life much more easily. It is important too, to try
and find new interests – hobbies – not just ways of filling in time,
like unnecessary cleaning or shopping, or working far too hard, like
Brenda above.

> In the ongoing flux of life, human beings undergo many
> changes. Arriving, departing, growing, declining, achieving,
> failing – every change involves a loss and a gain. The old
> environment must be given up, the new accepted.
>
> Stephen, 1998

Emotions which are in the grief group, such as despair, distress, a
sense of hopelessness, could be likened to 'lesser or little deaths'.
Events such as losing a job, children leaving home, losing a limb
are important 'griefs' to have to deal with and I would like to illustrate this with regard to the grief of losing a limb. There are still
new changes which have to be accepted, and the essential oils
would be chosen in the same way as grief through losing a loved
one.

CASE STORY

In France, when teaching Swiss Reflex Therapy, one of my students was a man called Fabien who had only one leg (from an accident two years previously, in which he had lost his hip as well). How was he going to participate in a course which involved treating two feet? When I began to talk to him, I could see that he was recovering remarkably well from the grief of losing a limb in the prime of his life and the many changes he must have had to make, both emotionally and physically. He was spending six weeks in a special centre to help him adjust to having had his bladder removed. His carer was a warm, positive person, who had taken an introductory course in aromatherapy with me two years previously and was already helping him with essential oils. However, she was certain that Swiss Reflex would help him to help himself.

We decided that although Fabien would learn how to do the treatment on the feet of other people, he would also learn how to use his hand reflexes for self-treatment. The class was most supportive, and by the end of the second day, each was happy to have him as a partner, doing one foot and the opposite hand, for balance. Only one lady seemed reluctant to accept the situation, but after giving her a mixture of basil and melissa to inhale deeply every hour *(see the oils for 'fear' below)*, she *offered* to have Fabien at the next changeover of partners!

The oils we used in the reflex cream for Fabien were:

- frankincense, to help his physical and mental pain and his depression
- sweet marjoram, to calm his fears about being with everyone, and for its neurotonic ability
- cypress, to relieve feelings of frustration at being unable to do all that he wanted, and to strengthen his nervous system.

The emotional change in Fabien was evident towards the end of the second afternoon, when, even allowing for the creation of group energy achieved by like-minded people meeting together for the first time, he began to smile and became much more relaxed than his carer had secretly hoped for. This was also due in part to the fact that the essential oils (and the treatment, of course) had relieved much of the pain which had been his constant companion since the accident – even with pain-killing drugs.

CASE STORY

Ellen, 69, had worked at the local baker's efficiently and loyally for 10 years. They were moving to a new shop and re-employed all the existing staff except Ellen, without even acknowledging her length of service. She was devastated, and on her way home called at my friend's aromatherapy clinic in floods of tears. Pouring out her story, she said 'Can you give me an essential oil to cheer me up?' Brenda knew that her husband had died the previous year, her mother, who had been her main comfort, dying unexpectedly six weeks later. Ellen had only missed one week at work at these times and confided that she didn't know what she would do at home now all day.

Brenda gave her frankincense and 'Shirley' lavender (which she loved) on a hanky, with a few drops of cypress and, knowing she was a conscientious worker, also offered her a job for three days a week. Ellen was overjoyed; she loved essential oils and had been given them for minor disorders before. She has since proved her worth and absolutely adores her job.

One day, Brenda's daughter (who is in charge of the clinic since Brenda's retirement), noticed Ellen was on edge and was chatting incessantly in a negative sort of way about nothing and getting on everyone's nerves. When Dawn spoke to her mother that night, Brenda remembered that the anniversary of Ellen's husband's death was in a few days. She suggested that Dawn put drops of cypress around the reception counter before Ellen arrived the next day. Cypress was chosen to increase Ellen's emotional stamina, and Dawn noticed that not only did she become more cheerful but the incessant chatter dried up after an hour and they had a super day at the shop. Both Dawn and Brenda realized later that this was no doubt due to the fact that cypress has astringent properties!

Essential Oils

Some of the essential oils which cope effectively with grief are the most costly ones and this is one instance in which choices should be made according to the depth of your grief. Grief is the cost of having loved – the deeper the love, the deeper the grief – and you are worth it, because *they* were (Stephen, 1998). The essential oils we need are those which

- relieve pain (analgesic)
- lift the spirits
- calm and sedate, as well as boost, the nervous system (balancing)
- have the capacity to heal, including bruises (cicatrizant)
- are a tonic to the heart
- stimulate the appetite
- stimulate the immune system
- stimulate the mind.

Frankincense *(Boswellia carteri)*

Although frankincense is not the most cited oil for supporting grief, it is, in my opinion, one of the most important oils to use. It is analgesic, relieving the mental pain associated with grief, especially in its early stages; it is energizing to the nervous system, thereby strengthening it against adversity, including distress; its cicatrizant (healing) qualities help to heal wounds (mental as well as physical); its antidepressant qualities revitalize and soothe the spirit. As it is also anti-inflammatory, it could be of use to those who feel some anger associated with their grief. According to Keville & Green (1995) and Mojay (1996), its calming effects will help to release the past and encourage tranquillity of mind, while Battaglia (1995) tells us that it slows the breathing, which suggests it would help allay fear of the future.

Marjoram *(Origanum majorana)*

This oil possesses a host of properties which are indispensable for coping with grief. It is a balancing oil like frankincense, strengthening and relaxing the nerves; it is analgesic, so can help relieve the pain of grief; its neurotonic properties suggest it will be effective on nervous depression, lifting the spirits and helping to deal with anguish and emotional exhaustion. It is calming, helping with any worries, agitation or irritability which may be experienced. According to most aromatherapy authors who write about the emotions, it relieves the feeling of loneliness, inevitable when one has lost the one nearest and dearest to you.

Lavender *(Lavandula angustifolia)*

Our old and valued friend, lavender, possesses many of the virtues which will be of help in relieving grief. It is analgesic, relieving the pain of grief; sedative, an invaluable aid for easing the stress of the situation and enabling the mind to relax, so that getting to sleep will be less difficult. Lavender is a tonic to the heart and its healing properties can help to heal any emotional wounds brought to the surface because of the bereavement; being also a tonic to the nervous system, it is effective should depression set in. As lavender is anti-inflammatory it can help disperse hurt or mental bruising, as well as being able to help release any angry or irritating thoughts which may be part of the hurting experience. Holmes (1992) tells us that it encourages acceptance of painful situations – and Lawless (1994) that it 'sweeps away grief'.

Sage *(Salvia officinalis)*

Sage oil contains thujone, and although the type of thujone in it has not been proved to be toxic, it is best to use this oil sparingly. Its analgesic properties suggest that it would help relieve the pain of grief; indeed, both Battaglia (1997 p.198) and Keville & Green (1995 p.67) cite it for grief. Like frankincense, it is also cicatrizant (healing). It is a decongestant, indicating that it may clear a mind which has become overcrowded with differing thoughts and emotions – and if anger is one of these, sage happens also to be antispasmodic, suggesting it will help relieve any anger spasms. It is neurotonic, so, like marjoram, it can lift the spirits and help dispel depression.

Cypress *(Cupressus sempervirens)*

Cypress is well-known for regulating the nervous system; it is therefore a balancing oil. Although it is not specific to grief, it is most useful for the 'ups and downs' which form part of grief. It also strengthens the nervous system, enabling it to reach a state of relaxation, whilst at the same time it may increase emotional resilience. It is antispasmodic, therefore can help reduce any feelings of irritability or frustration which may be part of the grieving process. Mojay (1996 p.67) writes that it dissolves remorse, which is a useful attribute in grief and that it is effective against fear, instilling optimism – an excellent feeling to aim for.

Melissa *(Melissa officinalis)*

Melissa is one of the most expensive essential oils, but is worth its price not only for its instant calming effect on the shock which may have begun the grieving process (best in synergy with clary sage and rosemary), but also for the help it can give to the 'side-effects' of grief. It is balancing, historically being known as an antidepressant, 'strengthening nature much in all its actions . . . it reviveth the heart . . . and driveth away all troublesome cares and thoughts out of the mind arising from melancholy' (Culpeper). Its sedative, calming effects indicate that it will help to cope with any restlessness, anxieties or worries associated with the grief being experienced, while its anti-inflammatory properties suggest that it could cool any anger or frustration which may be felt during the grieving process. The fact that it may restore clarity to a confused, dependent mind (Mojay) rounds off melissa's collection of attributes.

Neroli *(Citrus aurantium var. amara – flower)*

Like several of the above oils, neroli is antidepressive, and as it is also lightly tranquillizing, it is most useful for the emotional shock which begins the grieving process. It aids sleep and is neurotonic, helping to lift the spirits against inevitable fatigue. Its wonderful aroma seems to alleviate 'deep emotional pain which robs us of hope and joy' (Mojay 1996 p.101).

The essential oil from the leaves of the same tree, petitgrain *(Citrus aurantium var. amara – leaf)* is energizing to the nervous system, so could be helpful if cost is an important consideration in the choice of oils *(see Chapter 8)*.

Rose *(Rosa damascena, Rosa centifolia)*

Another oil to deplete your pocket, but a beautifully aromatic and balancing oil which is both relaxing and uplifting to the spirits and, as Fischer-Rizzi (1990) writes, brings joy to the heart. Its neurotonic and energizing properties help to lift the gloomy depression which is part of grief, helping also to cope with the mental fatigue associated with going over things again and again without being able to receive an answer. Like frankincense, it can heal psychological wounds, and according to Mojay (1996 p.113), it slows the breathing, which suggests it would help allay fear of what the future will now hold. It is anti-inflammatory, so can cool any hint of anger or other emotional stress which appears on the horizon.

Although the above oils are the major players, other oils have some of the physical properties needed to relieve grief:

- bergamot *(Citrus bergamia);* neurotonic, healing and sedative
- clove bud *(Syzygium aromaticum);* analgesic, healing, neurotonic and calming, immunostimulant
- geranium *(Pelargonium graveolens);* analgesic, neurotonic and healing
- niaouli *(Melaleuca viridiflora);* analgesic, neurotonic and immunostimulant
- rosemary *(Rosmarinus officinalis);* analgesic, neurotonic and healing
- sweet thyme *(Thymus vulgaris,* alcohol chemotype) cardiotonic, neurotonic and immunostimulant.

Anger

> Everyone should be quick to listen, but slow to speak and slow to become angry.
>
> James 1:19

> Do not let the sun go down while you are still angry.
>
> Ephesians 4:26

> A patient man has great understanding, but a quick tempered man displays his folly.
>
> Proverbs 14:29

Anger, Irritability, Impatience, Touchiness, Frustration

- anger
  hot displeasure, irritability, choler, bitterness, fury, ill temper,

rage, resentment, wrath, indignation, passion, hatred
- irritability
annoyance, impatience, touchiness, dyspepsia, displeasure, cantankerousness, indignation, resentment, wrath, exasperation
- touchiness
over-sensitivity, quick-temperedness, irritability, temperamental, churlish, cantankerous
- impatience
annoyance, intolerance, irritability, touchiness
- frustration
dissatisfied, disappointed, disheartened, upset, discouraged, thwarted, embittered, resentful

See how anger, touchiness and impatience all share irritability as a characteristic, annoyance being shared with both impatience and irritability. Anger, irritability and frustration all have resentment in their lists and although frustration, its feelings of bitterness with anger, in all other respects it fits better into the group of emotions characterized by grief. I think it is safe to say that being frustrated is one of the *causes* of anger and for that reason, I feel it has a place in this group.

It is interesting to note that bile (also called choler, which is in the anger line above), is 'a thick bitter fluid excreted from the liver, pertaining to irritability and ill-temper'; dyspeptic, in the irritability line above, means 'suffering from or pertaining to indigestion'. This suggests that essential oils to aid digestion – and, in particular, indigestion, would be a good choice for relieving anger and irritability.

Anger is one of the trickiest emotions to deal with and is often repressed; it usually ends up adversely affecting the lives of those expressing it frequently. To help correct negative anger, we have to be able to admit that we experience it. Having crossed this difficult bridge, it then takes positive thoughts, patience and time to change ourselves.

To rule one's anger is well; to prevent it is still better.

Tryon Edwards

There are many and varying degrees of anger, ranging from simple impatience or annoyance to fury or rage, an emotion which seems to be affecting some motorists nowadays, unfortunately! Apart from the difference in the severity of anger experienced, it can affect different people in different ways, depending on their personality, as well as the circumstances. It can also be addressed to oneself as well as to others. Not only that, but it can be justified – or unjustified. The use of the appropriate essential oils can calm those whose justified anger is aroused because of someone else's unjustified action – or help to bring peace to those whose anger is unjustified (inexcusable), although perhaps immediately regretted.

We are conditioned to think of anger as a negative, destructive emotion (which it frequently is), rather than a positive force for change (which it can sometimes be). We should also not forget that properly directed anger is a necessary, positively assertive and creative force and is only 'negative' when out of balance or control (Mojay, 1999 p.154).

CASE STORY

Three years ago a friend of mine was mugged and had to be given oxygen for five hours after the attack. The experience revived her dread of going out. She had suffered from agoraphobia for a long time before, and it had taken four years of treatment under a psychiatrist to recover fully. She was very angry that because of the mugging, she had to go through all the exercises again to prepare her mind for venturing out alone.

To help her control and dissipate this anger, she used cotton wool balls secreted in the top pocket of her dress, blouse or jacket with several drops of cypress and bergamot (these are beneficial both to anger and fear), adding to it a precious drop or two of rose otto for comfort (rose is an emotionally soothing oil). Although her husband won't let her go out unaccompanied since the mugging, her fear abated quicker than she thought and she was able to go back to work almost straight away, with abated anger!

Let's look at some different types of anger:

- instant, expressed anger
  usually in the form of words, which often ends in regret

- instant, unexpressed anger
  often relieved by involuntarily kicking something, or punching the nearest hard object; unfortunately, this can also hurt physically! Voluntary actions are preferable and are usually less painful, like slamming a door, punching a cushion or throwing a plate
- 'delayed' anger
  when we are sufficiently in control of our emotions not to express anger immediately; this can often be dissipated (released, vented) by an action like beating a doormat against the wall to remove the dust, scrubbing a floor, chopping wood, running round the block, etc., which brings about a release of feelings and has a sense of achievement as a side-effect, so satisfaction is also gained
- long-term repressed anger
  which can 'eat' into us and affect our mental as well as our physical health. If chronic anger is repeatedly 'fed' by angry thoughts, depression can develop:

> Indeed, when we stifle so-called negative emotions such as sadness or anger, we may become depressed and hopeless, which can be harmful to our health ... Once we acknowledge, express and resolve feelings such as sadness and anger, we are generally less likely to become depressed or hopeless.
>
> Domar & Dreher, 1997 p.159

When anger continues to boil inside, or rankle someone, it festers like an ulcer, which suggests that oils which help to heal physical ulcers would also heal emotional 'ulcers' ('rankle', believe it or not, is another word for ulcer). Deep anger should never be left to smoulder inside, or it can turn into resentment, bitterness – or even hatred, which is not good for the soul or the health. In fact, strong destructive emotions do just that – 'destroy' the body – and festering anger could well make you susceptible to stomach ulcers, kidney stones, etc.

> Anger is injurious to the liver ... the force of life of the body is interrupted and the blood rushes upwards and causes dizziness.
>
> Veith 1992

Although essential oils will help to release this inner anger, positive thinking and faith in what you can achieve are essential too, and can be practised while vaporizing relaxing essential oils. Think, too, about forgiveness (not easy I know); try forgiving whoever was the cause of feeling this way – this is the only thing which can heal the anger inside. You will be amazed at how much better you will feel if you keep saying 'I forgive him' or 'I forgive her', even if you don't really mean it at that precise moment in time. Repeated affirmations will eventually put you in the frame of mind where forgiveness becomes a reality – and you are healed *(see Chapter 4)*.

Dr Redford Williams, from the Behavioural Medicine Research Center in America, has been saying for years that having a hostile personality can kill us, most often by heart disease, but also by injuries and accidents. Anger speeds the heart rate, raises blood pressure and disrupts coronary arteries (McCasland, 1999).

Other emotions which may surface during the course of being cross or angry are:

- remorse, regret
  of having spoken angrily in haste
- guilt
  knowing that your unjustified anger or fury has hurt someone else
- frustration
  wanting to let out your anger, but not daring to, because you might lose your job
- fear
  of what might happen because, in your anger, you let out a secret with which you had been entrusted
- shock
  if the anger was against you and unjustified

Regarding essential oils, if any other emotion surfaces not in this group, just turn to the group in which it appears. For anger and its companion emotions, those which are calming and sedative would be the most helpful, and some oils have properties that would help release long-term anger, should this be a part of your problem. However, it is really up to you, once you can admit to having anger in your system or being easily aroused to it, to select those which suit your particular needs. Let us now have a look at the appropriate essential oils; we need those which:

- will sedate, calm and soothe
- will relax cramp and spasm (antispasmodic)
- are healing – including boils and ulcers (cicatrizant)
- relieve irritation and inflammation
- release inflammation-producing catarrh
- are analgesic (for anger against self).

Essential Oils

Roman chamomile *(Chamaemelum nobile)*

The calming, sedative properties of chamomile, coupled with being anti-inflammatory, make it a good choice for all emotions in this group, and as it is an appropriate oil for children, it is a great help to soothe their tantrums and bursts of temper. These same properties will help to soothe frustration or anger due to underlying stress. It is also healing to boils and ulcers (which are usually inflamed and irritable), which suggests its use for resolving irritations which otherwise may develop into a deeper form of anger, such as resentment, as well as healing the anger itself. Should anger reach this pitch, then the antispasmodic effect of chamomile comes into play, helping to relieve these feelings from their emotional 'cramp'. Finally, remembering the meaning of dyspeptic *(above)*, chamomile, as it is helpful to physical indigestion, would be appropriate also to ease the emotional 'indigestion' suffered with annoyance.

Bergamot *(Citrus bergamia)*

Bergamot is a calming, sedative oil with a pleasant, refreshing and uplifting aroma (children love it), and the sedative effect is particularly soothing when one is agitated (Price & Price, 1999 p.320). Being refreshing and uplifting suggests it could be an oil which could help you to forgive whoever was responsible for your anger, soothing this latter emotion at the same time. Its antispasmodic properties suggest it will release pent-up feelings and hidden anger that have been 'cramped' inside; indeed, according to Mojay (1996 p.53), it is especially useful to release unexpressed anger. He also suggests that bergamot promotes optimism – isn't that just what you need to help your positive thinking with regard to forgiveness! None of us like being angry, even if we don't want to admit we are bottling it up inside. Because bergamot is cicatrizant (healing) and eases indigestion, it seems natural to expect it to help heal anger and, whilst restoring normality to feelings ranging from annoyance to fury, to promote a forgiving feeling too.

Lavender *(Lavandula angustifolia)*

An oil with which everyone is familiar, lavender's sedative and calming properties, added to its antispasmodic and anti-inflammatory actions, will ease most of the emotional conditions in this group, its added analgesic properties helping the emotional pain of frustration or inner anger. Indeed, Holmes (1992) suggests that it encourages acceptance of a painful situation, which again could help if forgiveness is difficult, particularly as it is also cicatrizant, so may help to heal the disagreement as well as the feelings experienced. Several writers on aromatherapy suggest lavender for irritability. As it has an aroma with which many children are familiar, it is valuable (as is bergamot – they make a good synergy) in a situation where tantrums or temper show themselves.

Lemon *(Citrus limon)*

Lemon's calming and anti-inflammatory properties suggest it would be useful for most of the emotions in this group. The fact that it is antispasmodic and helps break up kidney stones and gallstones suggests its importance for anger or resentment which has become stony, or 'hard', inside. Being anti-inflammatory both for boils and stomach ulcers suggests its efficiency to deal not only with anger, but possibly rage and fury as well. It has an uplifting aroma, which suggests that, like bergamot, it would be helpful in situations where children are involved. Mojay (1996 p.92) tells us it 'clears heat' and Battaglia (1997 p.175) recommends it when 'hot and bothered', which can be part and parcel of the emotions in this group.

Geranium *(Pelargonium graveolens)*

Yet another antispasmodic, anti-inflammatory oil, geranium is also cicatrizant (healing) and analgesic – which suggests it to be a most useful oil for most of the emotions in this group, especially where anger or any of its subsidiaries has resulted in resentment or hatred, both of which have need of a healing touch, not only for the sake of the person expressing the anger, but also for the one on the receiving end. Price & Price (1999 pp.337–8) tell us that its calming properties soothe agitation, which, added to its analgesic properties, will help the emotional pain of frustration or inner anger, encouraging acceptance of a painful situation and promoting forgiveness. Its cicatrizant ability may also help to heal the disagreement. Its neurotonic properties will help alleviate frustration where anger is combined with disappointment or despair.

Rosemary *(Rosmarinus officinalis)*
The properties of rosemary which help the emotions in this group are mostly the same as those for geranium: cicatrizant, antispasmodic, anti-inflammatory, neurotonic. However, each has an extra property that the other hasn't got; rosemary, unlike geranium, does not relieve indigestion, but it has the ability, like lemon, to break up gallstones, which suggests its importance for alleviating anger or resentment which has become like stone inside the mind. It may not be calming, but its undisputed power to clarify the mind and stimulate the brain may provide the mental strength to deal with anger aimed at ourselves – and save us from unnecessary and possibly hurtful retaliation which we may afterwards regret. Fischer-Rizzi (1990 p.160) says that it gives strength against strong emotions – and anger is certainly one of those!

Peppermint *(Mentha x piperita)*
Peppermint is anti-inflammatory and excellent for bringing down a fever, both of which properties suggest its usefulness in relieving the heat produced in an angry situation. It is also antispasmodic, suggesting its ability to unblock hidden anger or resentment. Although it is not calming to the nervous system, it is soothing to red, inflamed, irritated skin which suggests that it will soothe and reduce any emotions in this group which would make one hot, annoyed or irritable.

Although the above are the major players, several other oils have some of the physical properties which will relieve anger:

- basil *(Ocimum basilicum);* analgesic, antispasmodic, stimulating to the digestion
- cypress; antispasmodic and calming (regulates the sympathetic nervous system and reduces irritation)
- coriander *(Coriandrum sativum);* analgesic, anti-inflammatory, antispasmodic and helpful to indigestion
- mandarin *(Citrus reticulata);* a strong sedative, antispasmodic
- marjoram *(Origanum majorana);* analgesic, antispasmodic, expectorant (releasing catarrh)
- melissa *(Melissa officinalis);* anti-inflammatory, antispasmodic, calming and sedative and soothing to indigestion
- niaouli *(Melaleuca viridiflora);* anti-inflammatory, healing to boils and ulcers and valuable in breaking down gallstones
- ylang ylang *(Cananga odorata);* antispasmodic and sedative.

Fear

> The man who fears suffering is already suffering from what he fears.
>
> Michel de Montaigne

Fear, Apprehension, Trepidation, Dismay, Dread, Terror, Panic

- fear
  apprehension, anxiety, trepidation, dismay, dread, terror, panic
- apprehension
  fear, alarm, anxiety, doubt, dread, mistrust
- trepidation
  alarm, apprehension, agitation, dread, fear, panic
- dismay
  agitation, alarm, anxiety, apprehension, dread, fear
- dread
  fear, alarm, apprehension, dismay, fear, terror.

Three of the emotions above (trepidation, dismay and dread) share apprehension with the basic emotion of this group, namely fear; dismay and trepidation share the feeling of agitation. Anxiety is central to most of the expressions of fear and if it is present in your own experience, when selecting oils, refer to those on the anxiety list in the previous chapter. Fear can also be a painful (and perhaps harmful) emotion, depending on its intensity and duration.

> If a man harbours any sort of fear, it percolates through all his thinking, damages his personality, makes him landlord to a ghost.
>
> Lloyd Douglas

Fear is a necessary emotion which was originally essential for self-preservation, and still is occasionally, but in modern times it is not always 'frightening' as we understand the word; it can even be stimulating if you are a rock climber whose fear is an exhilarating experience! It depends mostly on the situation, and also on the personality of the individual. Watching someone else's fear on television will affect each of us differently; some may experience fear themselves quite strongly, while others may feel nothing more than a little apprehensive about what will happen next.

Fear is a little like grief in that it can involve more than one emotion, for example:

- guilt can bring on fear of being found out
- anger can bring on fear of losing your job after having lost your temper
- lack of confidence, a kind of 'fear' in itself, can bring on the true fear of having made the wrong decision.

So when selecting essential oils, these points need to be taken into account. Also,

> fear and rejection always tend to be present when people are challenged by something new or unknown, and this is usually accompanied by an unexamined presumption that what we have already achieved will be somehow undermined, devalued or diminished.
>
> Eccles, 1995

The emotion of fear can manifest itself in several strengths; from a forthcoming exam or performance, which can fill you with apprehension or dread, to the immense fear experienced after being told you have cancer, which involves terror and panic, in fact, practically all the emotions in this group.

A human being's most basic need is food; indeed, stone-age man was willing to risk being killed by wild animals in order to get food. The next basic need is safety, fear being the emotion which is aroused by lack of it. Being alone in a large or old house or in a dark wood can be frightening; harmless snakes, mice and, for some people, even spiders can induce a feeling of terror. Incidentally, courage is not the absence of fear; perseverance, despite the fear, is the essence of courage (Chance, 1998).

Many people choose a job that gives them security and safety. They save money against possible future bad times and hoard medicaments sometimes to the point of hypochondria (like the story of my mother in Chapter 2) – all to allay the emotion of fear.

Stress and fear are closely related. Under stress, fear can often manifest itself. Similarly, when frightened for any length of time, stress is also present. However, if relating fear to the three stages involved in stress *(see previous chapter)*, fear usually only reaches the third stage if it is deeply embedded and long-lasting, like knowing you have cancer or living with a man of whom you are terrified, but cannot leave. The first stage is exactly the same as that of stress, where, when the fear is first experienced, energy and extra adrenalin are released (among other physical changes within the body), to give extra strength and resources for any action needed to save the situation.

We all suffer from fear in some shape or form, not necessarily in conscious fear, but in the interplay of our body–mind relationship, both in health and in sickness ... Fear is created by the surplus energy arising from a threatening situation and if that energy can be let out in action, that is good ... Imagine primitive man in his cave, with his mate and young ones. The snarl of the sabre toothed tiger awakens him – and immediately the speed of his heartbeat is increased, so his breathing quickens and deepens, his blood pressure rises and the liver is stimulated to pour out more sugar into the blood. In this way, his muscles have adequate supplies of energy to cope with the needs of the situation. At the same time, two little glands above the kidneys (the adrenal glands) pour into the blood a chemical called adrenalin. This has an immediate action on the nerve endings, which become sensitized and those nerves which control the pupils of his eyes cause these to dilate, which considerably enlarges his field of vision, in preparation for his escape.

Robinson, 1948

The above was written by my father for a lecture he gave to the Psychological Society in Newcastle, when I was just a teenager. I am quite impressed that his explanation is the same as the first stage of stress expressed in the earliest book I can find on the subject; his information, I believe, came from the great psychologist, Jung.

We should not be ashamed of our fear; we need to recognize that it is part of our nature and just needs to be coped with in a way that will not jeopardise our health. If you can verbalize your fears with a trusted friend, a lot of the underlying tension will be taken away (you can share your friend's fears as well). We have to accept that a certain amount of fear is going to manifest itself when we start a new job, fly for the first time or try to accomplish something difficult, so repeat positive phrases, like 'I am in control of my fear', 'I am perfectly calm', 'I am not afraid of . . . '. Use essential oils in advance as well as during the situation itself, and you will be surprised at how much your fear will be diminished.

Fear can also be experienced due to a horrendous event, like being viciously attacked or raped. An aromatherapist friend and teacher told me about a client of hers:

CASE STORY

Lilian came to Barbara through a friend, suffering from panic attacks. Some time ago she had been raped in her own home by an intruder and she was now afraid of everything and everybody. Every time she tried to go out alone she had a panic attack and had to go back. She was also angry, because the perpetrator had never been brought to justice. She could not bear anyone to touch her, so

Barbara offered her help through inhalation alone. She gave her a tiny bottle of melissa and explained that every time she felt her fear or panic coming on she should take off the lid and inhale deeply. The client loved the aroma, which was fortunate, as this would contribute to its effectiveness. Barbara also offered a listening ear if she would like to talk about how she felt, telling her that this would help to relieve her feelings and to expel the horrendous experience from her mind. The young lady took her up on this offer and made rapid progress over the next six months, even allowing Barbara to massage her hands and feet after a few weeks.

She has now completely recovered from her panic attacks, and her emotions and thoughts have returned to a more balanced and accepting state, so much so, that within four years she was happily married.

Let's look at the oils now which will help you to diminish or face your fears. Depending on the kind of fear experienced, you will need to select those oils which apply to your particular fear, the choice being from oils which

- are calming and soothing
- are stimulating to the mind
- relieve spasm
- slow down the heartbeat
- act as a tonic to, and therefore strengthen, the heart
- reduce blood pressure
- are a tonic to the respiratory system
- stimulate the digestion (including the liver)
- strengthen the kidneys
- relieve nausea
- normalize diarrhoea
- are analgesic.

Essential Oils

Basil *(Ocimum basilicum)*
An oil which fulfils many of the criteria above is basil. It has a traditional reputation for easing nervous disorders, and Gerard (1545–

1611) said that it makes the heart merry and glad. This, together with the fact that it is cardiotonic, suggests it would be ideal to set a heart depressed with strong emotions of fear onto a healing path. Dread and trepidation can start the heart pumping madly, so basil's ability to slow down a heart which is beating too fast makes it useful prior to exams, job interviews, etc. Basil is a mental stimulant, suggesting it will help clear and strengthen the mind in situations such as dread or terror, helping to restore composure and serenity; this clearing effect also indicates that it may help clear doubt or indecision if these are part of the emotion being experienced. Its antispasmodic effects on both the digestive system and the muscles which control movement of the body and limbs render it useful for relaxing the whole body when fear has made it tense. The fact that it is analgesic suggests its ability to soothe any pain connected with the fear being experienced. It stimulates the digestive system as a whole, revitalizing it, which is a great help when fear has affected it adversely. As it is also effective against nausea it will soothe the 'sick' feeling often associated with fear.

Melissa *(Melissa officinalis)*

Although one of the more costly oils, melissa has many qualities which help dispel fears of all kinds, plus it has an exceptional aroma, which has a positive effect on most women. It lowers the blood pressure and has both a calming and a sedative action, all of which suggest that it would be particularly effective for anyone experiencing panic or terror, or whose blood pressure is already high. The sedative and calming properties of melissa make it invaluable for ongoing fear, nervous agitation or apprehension, and if sleep is difficult at this time, it will help induce sleep. Before a worrying event, such as exams, a visit to the dentist or admission into hospital, apprehension makes the heart beat faster and as melissa is indicated for normalizing a rapid heartbeat, it will soothe the apprehension and dread being experienced. Because the digestive system doesn't work at its best during an ongoing fear situation, some people may experience nervous indigestion. Melissa is antispasmodic, especially to the digestive system, so it is doubly effective here, relaxing those muscles involved; as it is indicated for nausea it can also relieve that 'sick' feeling in the stomach.

Marjoram *(Origanum majorana)*

Marjoram is a calming oil to the nervous system and is particularly useful if fear is preventing sleep. It relaxes nervous spasm, which suggests it can release the tight feeling in the chest which is often a symptom of fear, relieving also any pain connected with this feeling, as it is analgesic too. It is a respiratory tonic, so can help slow down the rapid breathing which is evident in the early stages. The fact that it is a heart tonic and relieves both tachycardia and palpitations implies that it will calm and regulate the heartbeat; its ability to lower blood pressure is also of importance here. Add to this its very competent antispasmodic effects on muscles, the respiratory system and nerves and it would seem that the sum total of its relaxing effects on any stress connected with ongoing fear is very great. One of its assets is the ability to reduce sweating, which, as this is often one of the symptoms of fear, would be a suitable oil to use, even if one is only sweating emotionally, so to speak. Last but not least, marjoram happens to be a tonic to the nerves, so should help to instil courage where there is apprehension or dread.

Bergamot *(Citrus bergamia)*

Bergamot, like melissa, is both calming and sedative to the nervous system, making it ideal for chronic fear symptoms. At the same time, it is neurotonic, suggesting its use not only to relax the fear but also to give the necessary courage to face the situation, as with marjoram. The aroma alone is uplifting, which is an asset for anyone whose fear is making them depressed. It is antispasmodic, relaxing any tension which may be present. As the digestive system slows down when fear takes hold, and bergamot is a digestive stimulant and good for nervous indigestion, this suggests it will be a beneficial oil for fear symptoms, even if long-term. Rovesti, a well-known professor at an Italian university, conducted research with essential oils at several psychiatric clinics and has described the effects of bergamot in relieving fear and anxiety (cited in Fischer-Rizzi, 1990 p.72).

Lavender *(Lavandula officinalis)*

Lavender, although it has no digestive properties which will help allay fear, has nevertheless several useful properties to help other aspects of this emotion. It is well known for its calming and sedative properties and is also used for reducing blood pressure, often heightened during fear. Its relaxing properties include the ability to aid sleep if insomnia is one of the presenting symptoms in connection with the aspect of fear experienced. It is cardiotonic and this, together with its neurotonic properties, suggests it will help boost courage at a time when apprehension, dread or sheer fear have taken hold. It is antispasmodic, like all the oils so far mentioned, which would help release the muscle tension associated with fear, while its analgesic properties suggest its ability to ease any pain suffered as a result of the fear.

Rosemary *(Rosmarinus officinalis)*

Although rosemary is neither calming nor sedative, it is cardiotonic and relieves palpitations, which will help return an over-fast heartbeat to normal. Mojay (1996 p.115) confirms this when he says that rosemary strengthens the heartbeat – just what is needed when in a fearful state. The fact that rosemary is a mental stimulant suggests it will help strengthen the mind too, especially if dread or terror enter the fear picture; its mind-clearing effect may also help clear doubt or indecision if these are present. Rosemary is antispasmodic, especially on muscles, which makes it particularly effective to relax the tightness typically experienced in most categories of fear; its analgesic properties suggest it will help any mental pain being suffered at the same time. It is a good digestive oil, being a stimulant as well as relieving indigestion – particularly painful indigestion, which indicates (together with its analgesic ability) that it would efficiently help any pain connected with the fear.

Ylang ylang *(Cananga odorata)*

The calming and sedative properties of ylang ylang make it appropriate for chronic fear symptoms, especially as it not only slows down a rapid heartbeat but is also effective in lowering the blood pressure, which may rise in certain people when experiencing fear. It is antispasmodic, like all the oils recommended above, which suggests it will relax spasms of fear, as its skills in this respect are mainly to do with the digestive system, which is adversely affected during the emotion of fear.

Although the above oils are the major players, several other oils have some of the physical properties which will help relieve fear:

- lemon *(Citrus limon);* antispasmodic, astringent (diarrhoea), calming, reduces blood pressure
- cypress *(Cupressus sempervirens);* antispasmodic, calming, neurotonic and reduces sweating (increases emotional stamina – Keville & Green 1995 p.53)
- clary *(Salvia sclarea);* antispasmodic, calming to the nervous system, relieves diarrhoea
- sandalwood *(Santalum album);* astringent (diarrhoea), cardiotonic, nerve relaxant, sedative, general tonic
- geranium *(Pelargonium graveolens);* antispasmodic, analgesic, astringent (diarrhoea), calming
- rose otto *(Rosa damascena);* calming – though the aroma alone may help dispel deep-rooted fear.

Jealousy

> O! beware, my lord, of jealousy;
> it is the green-eyed monster which doth mock
> the meat it feeds on.
>
> William Shakespeare, Othello

Jealousy, Envy

- jealousy
  envy, covetousness, resentment (anger), intolerance, rivalry
- envy
  covetousness, craving, discontent, jealousy, resentment
- discontent
  unhappiness, resentment, annoyance, envy, yearning, displeasure, dissatisfaction
- desire
  yearning, covetousness, craving, want

The following emotions are linked:
- spite
  hatred, grudge, malice, rancour, bitterness

- suspicion
  mistrust, doubt

Jealousy and envy, rarely experienced on their own, are usually accompanied by other feelings or emotions. Apart from 'jealously' guarding a secret, or being normally 'jealous' about one's partner, most jealous feelings, like those of envy, are negative, destructive and hostile. Jealousy is often linked with anger and resentment and can, in certain circumstances, lead to passionate fury which could end in violence of some kind. Envy is less volatile and desire (mostly innocent) and discontent are emotions which can develop into one of the other two, given the circumstances.

> A heart at peace gives life to the body,
> but envy rots the bones.
>
> Proverbs 14:30

Jealousy can be caused by:
- inability to share
  usually possessions when we are young; in later life this includes people
- desire
  a craving for things or people or holidays that you, unlike your friends, cannot have
- unfulfilled ambition
  but your friend was successful in the same field
- dissatisfaction
  with what you have
- an over-suspicious mind
  looking furtively through your partner's pockets.

All but the last two can equally cause envy, which, although it may not cause anger, can certainly cause resentment and a feeling of being unable to let go and accept what we are lucky enough to have already. Let's see now where the similarities lie between the first four emotions: all but discontent have an element of covetousness and all but desire share resentment.

In jealousy, there is more of self-love than love of another.

François de la Rochefoucauld

It may be difficult to admit to being jealous or envious of another person or their possessions; however, once we can admit to it, we realize that it is a very destructive emotion; we stand to hurt not only ourselves but others as well. Some people:

> isolate themselves because they are jealous of friends who seem to have things they desire. They don't want to be around women who have advanced further in their careers, who appear to have conflict-free partnerships, or who possess some physical characteristic they covet.
>
> Domar & Dreher, 1997 p.141

If this applies to you, it's time to restructure your thinking! Would you really like to 'swap' with your friend? There is bound to be something you have which she hasn't – and if it had to be all or nothing, logical thinking would probably reveal that you are better off as you are. If you use positive thinking, you can learn to accept your friend's apparent advantages and be thankful for those you already have. Whatever others have – big car, bigger salary, better house or whatever – has no real impact on your life; it is all in your mind and can only harm you.

As I said earlier, other emotions can enter the picture of jealousy and its hostile associates. Let's look at them:

- anger and irritation
  which can surface in situations where your partner prefers his mother's cooking. She is a good cook, so you are jealous of her, but angry with your partner
- fear
  of what will happen if your partner eventually prefers, and goes off with, a mutual friend
- hatred
  of someone who always manages to get all the things you want – but cannot afford

- anxiety

  that someone else will be chosen for the job you want, especially
  if you know the person and he/she is more qualified than you are
- insecurity

  for the same reasons as fear and anxiety above.

CASE STORY

The aunt of a dear friend of mine developed cancer a few years ago.
She had an excellent job as financial secretary to a large firm and was
a very matter of fact, class-conscious, sometimes rather abrupt,
person. A few months ago, we were talking about emotions because I
was about to start writing this book. After asking after my friend's
aunt, as usual, I enquired if she had ever harboured any destructive
emotions, like resentment, jealousy or anger, or if she had been a
critical type of person, as these attributes often result in cancer (Hay,
1987). The story he told astonished me, as she had had a very successful career, had seemed content whenever I had seen her and was
not short of money:

She and her sister used to look after their invalid mother, but one
day her sister got married, and Auntie Ella never forgave her for
leaving her on her own, not only to cope, but also because it put
paid to any chance of her getting married herself. She resented her
father, who had not allowed her to go to university and she had
always criticized my friend's father (her brother), whom she insisted
had 'married beneath him'. Paul, her brother's other son, loved his
dad, but Auntie Ella was always complaining to Paul about him and
ended up not speaking to her nephew. My friend John, who is a sin-
cere Christian, sent a copy of Corinthians 1:13 to her, with a plead-
ing letter, but to no avail; she refused to contact Paul.

As I listened to this incredibly negative story about the life of a
woman I had respected, I realized that it was no wonder she had
developed cancer. I had recently been sending her essential oils for
her arthritis, at John's request, which she had found beneficial, and
juniper and rosemary were in this blend. Rosemary is beneficial to
both the emotions Ella had been harbouring for years (juniper benefiting the jealousy) so I wanted next time to send a new formula to
her to help dissipate the emotions which had destroyed her life. For

them to be completely successful, she would need to admit to having experienced – indeed, be still experiencing – destructive emotions before the essential oils could be expected to help after such a long period of resentment and jealousy. At the time of writing, Ella has only had the new mix for three weeks (in which I have substituted lemon – beneficial to both her emotional states – for the two other oils, which were specifically for arthritis), so I cannot say yet whether or not it has made any difference – I can only hope!

The essential oil properties which I feel will help to deal with jealousy and envy (and will automatically cover lesser emotions in this group) are those which are detoxifying and antifungal or antiviral. Jealousy and envy are like toxins in the mind, and fungal and viral infections are something which 'devour' a person, just like these two emotions. Antibacterial oils may also help, as bacteria are an unwanted invasion into our being, just like jealousy. Neurotonic properties may also help by stimulating the nervous system into a state of normality. Others may help too, and the complete list of properties from which oils can be chosen for individual feelings and reactions are:

• antibacterial
• antifungal
• antiviral
• detoxifying and cleansing to the whole system
• cicatrizant (healing)
• lytholitic (breaking down stones)
• anticatarrhal (clearing congestion).

Essential oils

Rosemary *(Rosmarinus officinalis)*
Rosemary excels itself with properties which I feel can help jealousy. It is detoxifying to the liver and gall bladder, which encourages one to hope that it could also detoxify the mind. It also helps dissolve gallstones, which again, could help dissolve the hardness of jealousy from the mind. Rosemary has other useful properties, such as antiviral, antifungal and anticatarrhal, which imply that it would be a valuable aid to ridding the mind of disagreeable emotions 'feeding' on

our better selves. It has the advantage of being cicatrizant (healing) too, and an emotion like jealousy certainly needs healing. We already know that rosemary is helpful in assuaging anger and its related emotions because of its healing, antispasmodic and anti-inflammatory properties, the latter property also rendering it effective against fear, if either of these emotions are experienced with the envy or jealousy.

Juniper *(Juniperus communis)*
Juniper is a well-known detoxicant to the kidneys and the digestive system as a whole, which suggests its suitability to get rid of jealousy. It also has the capacity to break down stones in the kidneys, which indicates that it can break down any hard, set feelings we may have, making them easier to be passed out of our minds. Juniper's diuretic and decongestant properties, which carry away excess fluid (including any toxins) via the kidneys and the lymph, suggest that it may help to release jealous feelings from our system; its ability to rid the system of catarrh may well do the same thing. If insomnia is a problem at the same time, juniper induces sleep. If anger or irritation forms an integral part of your jealousy, juniper's anti-inflammatory properties will help relieve these. Davis (1991) and Mojay (1996 p.87) both agree that juniper clears accumulated negative energy, which confirms its possible ability to clear both jealousy and anger from the mind.

Basil *(Ocimum basilicum)*
As basil is antiviral and antifungal, it could rid the mind of the symptoms of jealousy and envy which are eating into our system. It has the ability to help heal stomach ulcers, which may indicate its use in the milder forms of these unwanted emotions. Its antispasmodic and anti-inflammatory properties should help relieve any anger apparent at the same time, the former supporting any fear symptoms present also. As it is a mental stimulant and cardiotonic, one would hope it would strengthen both the heart and the mind and encourage the latter to think clearly about how jealousy may be adversely affecting the health. According to Keville & Green (1995 p.46), basil is another oil which helps clear negative thoughts.

Bergamot *(Citrus bergamia)*
As well as being antiviral and healing, bergamot has a refreshing,

uplifting smell. It is a calming and sedative oil, which could be useful, together with its healing properties, if unexpressed anger, resentment or stress show themselves with jealousy. Bergamot's anti-spasmodic properties will help release the anger, and if there is any fear connected with your jealousy, bergamot can help dispel this too. Where there are deep ongoing feelings of jealousy, or if envy has become a habit, causing depression, bergamot's neurotonic properties come into play to lift the spirits, whilst the sedative properties placate the emotions which are bothering you, helping to release pent-up feelings.

Lemon *(Citrus limon)*

Being an oil with many beneficial properties, lemon can help, not only with all aspects in the jealousy group, but with some of the emotions which can surface with them. It is capable of clearing both viruses and fungal infections, intimating its worth to help clear the mind of these worthless emotions. It also helps dissolve kidney stones, which implies it could help dissolve the stony hostile feeling of jealousy from our minds. Regarding accompanying emotions, lemon is anti-inflammatory and antispasmodic, both of which relieve emotions in the anger group; this effect is enhanced by its healing ability on boils and ulcers and its astringent qualities, which also will help anger. Lemon is a calming oil, which, together with the fact that it is a tonic to the heart and relieves nervous vomiting, would be an impeccable choice when fear enters the jealousy picture.

A few other oils have some of the physical properties which will help curtail jealousy and its attendant emotions:

- pine *(Pinus sylvestris);* antibacterial, antifungal, purifying, sweat-reducing (fear), anti-inflammatory (anger)
- sweet thyme *(Thymus vulgaris,* alcohol chemotype); antifungal, antiviral, cardiotonic (fear), antispasmodic and anti-inflammatory (anger).
- geranium *(Pelargonium graveolens);* antibacterial, antifungal, digestive stimulant (fear), antispasmodic (fear and anger), anti-inflammatory (anger), healing
- peppermint *(Mentha x piperita);* antibacterial, antifungal,

antiviral, decongestant, catarrh-reducing, digestive stimulant (fear), antispasmodic (fear and anger, anti-inflammatory (anger).

Guilt

Every man is guilty of the good he didn't do.

Voltaire

Guilt, Remorse, Regret, Shame

- guilt
  fear of disgrace, self-reproach, shame; usually brings regret, remorse, contrition
- remorse
  anguish, contrition, grief, guilt, regret, shame
- regret
  contrition, remorse, sorrow
- shame
  guilt, contrition, remorse, fear of disgrace, humiliation.

According to an international study from Associates for Research into the Science of Enjoyment, guilt is a British disease which could be threatening the nation's health. Apparently, 41 per cent of people in the UK would enjoy everyday pleasures more if they did not feel guilty. It is claimed that needless guilt reduces the stress-relieving and immune-system-boosting effects of enjoyment. The researchers covered eight countries and thirteen pleasures, including drinking wine, eating chocolates, sex and watching TV (cited in *Reader's Digest*, 1997).

Guilt (and its fellow feelings) is an unfortunate, complicated and difficult emotion. It only affects those who have a conscience about deceitful, unethical deeds they may have done, or hurtful, wounding words they may have spoken, perhaps in haste – and regretted almost immediately.

Every guilty person is his own hangman.

Seneca

Guilt can also begin to fester because of unfulfilled ambitions, with a feeling of having 'let the side down' (usually loved ones who expected more of you). It may even emerge because of forgetting to do something important, or of doing something for which you think you will be blamed later. Anxiety, often in the form of fear of the consequences, normally accompanies the emotions in this group.

It is difficult to select associated feelings from the explanations in the lists because, for example, guilt isn't remorse *per se,* though the latter usually follows almost immediately after the act – be it word or deed or even thought! Contrition appears in all interpretations of guilt, remorse being linked with regret and shame – shame being a part of both guilt and remorse. Sorrow and grief are connected with remorse and regret, but whichever feeling is experienced in this group, I feel that the group as a whole spell sorrow and grief.

Some forms of guilt include pain, especially after having done something perhaps unintentional but harmful to another person, such as causing a car accident, or being responsible for someone losing their job because of something you said. You may also feel sick, and you will certainly need uplifting in practically every application of the basic emotion.

One form guilt can take is when it is directed at yourself, for example, feeling guilty because you have taken time out of your busy day, with many commitments, for yourself; perhaps you went shopping and bought a new blouse or just a lipstick. Guilt such as this is often linked with not valuing yourself enough, living for the family at the expense of your own emotions, feeling guilty because you eat too much and are fat, but feel you can't help it. This kind of guilt is linked to shame; for example, when a woman is told she cannot conceive, she feels guilty (because of her husband's feelings) and she also experiences a certain amount of shame (Domar & Dreher, p.154).

Shame is more usually a feeling experienced after having done something which is regrettable in one's own eyes or in those of other people, and only surfaces 'as a result of someone else's judgement' (Lindenfield, 1997 p.119). It can also be experienced because of someone else's *action,* like telling your friends (when your child is within hearing) that 'Emily is so fat – I dread buying clothes for her' or making a child admit to wrongdoing in front of the whole class.

Sadly, particularly in the first case, such actions can drastically reduce any feeling of confidence the child may have had.

Some of the strongest feelings connected with guilt (and sometimes shame) are often associated with divorce, such as guilt over the happy times you had with your partner. If you have children, you may feel guilty about having disrupted their lives and shame because you feel you have put your happiness before theirs. Guilt feelings can also emerge connected to parents; not visiting them as often as you should or wishing you weren't there when you *do* go, especially if they are ill and you don't know what to say or do to pass the time.

Being driven by guilt can put you in a continual state of conflict. For example, occasionally when I accept a lecture tour abroad, I feel guilty, because I feel I ought to accept, though while I am accepting (with a smile), sometimes I don't really want to say yes. More often than not I have to cancel something nice, like a wedding, or a visit to friends. Whichever choice I make, I feel guilty! The following was in *The Aromatherapist* (1998), courtesy of *Candis* magazine:

How guilt ridden are you? Do you:
• suspect you'll have to pay the price for the times when you enjoy yourself
• often feel ashamed of things you've done?
• fear you don't deserve affection from those close to you?
• apologise for things which aren't your fault?
• often find yourself helping others when you don't want to/haven't really time?
• ever wish your conscience would leave you alone?
• feel a strong urge to confess things as soon as you've done them?
• sometimes think you've disappointed your parents by the life you've led?

If you've answered 'yes' to every question, you need to stop chiding yourself and start recognising your own needs.

If you are particularly vulnerable to guilt feelings, don't lose hope! Positive thinking is an excellent aid to making you feel better, and with essential oils in addition, the strength of your feelings can diminish, making them at least bearable, and at most able to change your attitude to life. This would result in fewer actions or words which may hurt others, leaving you less likely to be suffering the emotional consequences.

And now, let's investigate the essential oils which could help dissipate guilt. The physical properties which should be helpful are those which are:

- analgesic
- decongestant
- cicatrizant (healing)
- beneficial to nausea.
- detoxifying
- beneficial to indigestion
- cardiotonic (including palpitations)

You may also need to refer back to the essential oils which help anger, fear or grief, if these are in your emotional experience, though not the main cause for concern; these are mentioned briefly in the profiles of the oils below, where the required effect is also a property of that oil.

Essential Oils

Rosemary *(Rosmarinus officinalis)*
Rosemary has a great number of properties which are useful to the emotions in this group. It is detoxifying, which suggests its use after deliberate, unregretted, actions or words. If mental pain is present, rosemary's analgesic property should give some relief, and if your mind is blocked with mixed emotions which seem to have 'stuck', its decongestant action together with its effect on indigestion may help (Mojay (1996 p.115) recommends it for 'over thinking'). When long-standing guilt is causing depression, rosemary's cardiotonic action should strengthen the heart, and its neurotonic effect together with the fact that it is a mental stimulant suggest it will uplift and revive, giving clarity and energy to work out the best solution to resolve the situation. At the same time, rosemary, being cicatrizant, should begin a healing process, especially where contrition and shame are involved, and/or if grief is connected with the guilt feeling.

Lavender *(Lavandula angustifolia)*
Lavender is well known for its healing properties, which suggest that

it would be a good choice for conditions brought about by guilt, such as regret, remorse and contrition, helping to heal any anguish of mind and self-reproach at the same time. Used physically for scar tissue, it should help healing where guilt is deep inside; for example, when it is connected with grief. According to Holmes (1992), it encourages acceptance of a painful situation. Being analgesic, lavender should prove to be a useful oil where mental pain is part of the guilt feeling; it could also be useful if the emotion is getting you down, as it is a general tonic and its cardiotonic action will give you a boost. Should you be losing sleep because of over-worrying about the situation you are in, lavender is a favourite for insomnia.

Frankincense *(Boswellia carteri)*
A strong healing oil, invaluable for softening and renewing scar tissue, frankincense should prove its worth for healing all the emotions in the guilt 'family'. Being analgesic, it can help dissipate any mental pain being suffered and, if dejected or despondent, it will uplift the spirits at the same time with its antidepressive and energizing action. An immunostimulant, it will be of great use if you are already low in health, or long-standing guilt has begun to affect your health and you find yourself succumbing regularly to minor infections. If you are angry with yourself because of what you have done, remember frankincense is anti-inflammatory, suggesting its competence also to relieve the inflammation of your anger.

Peppermint *(Mentha x piperita)*
Peppermint is a good digestive oil, not only helping to relieve indigestion, but also alleviating nervous nausea and pains in the digestive tract. Its analgesic properties help in this respect as well, suggesting its ability to comfort guilt feelings causing emotional pain. It is decongestant, and as it is also a mental stimulant, aiding concentration, it should help clear congested minds of conflicting thoughts and mixed emotions. Indeed, Keville & Green (1995 p.65) tells us it 'clears mental fogginess'. If fear of the consequences of your actions is troubling you, peppermint's capacity to relieve nausea and nervous vomiting will be of value to those whose actions are making them feel sick. Should anger be strongly featured (perhaps if trying to cover up or deny the truth), peppermint is both antispasmodic and

anti-inflammatory, indicating its ability to calm hot anger spasms.
Other oils which may help with the emotions in this group are:

- geranium *(Pelargonium graveolens);* healing, analgesic and
  decongestant
- basil *(Ocimum basilicum);* cardiotonic, analgesic and
  decongestant
- pine *(Pinus sylvestris);* analgesic, decongestant, air purifier
- sandalwood *(Santalum album);* cardiotonic, decongestant.

Apathy

Apathy, Lethargy, Listlessness, Boredom

- apathy
  lack of feeling or interest, unconcern, indifference, inert,
  detached, unenthusiastic, unambitious, unemotional, inactive
- lethargy
  unnaturally sleepy or drowsy, inactive, languor, sluggishness,
  inertness (apathy), lack of energy, lack of concentration and
  interest, listlessness
- listlessness
  weariness, lack of interest, languor, inertia, sluggishness, lethargy,
  apathy
- boredom
  apathy, dullness, lethargy, lack of interest, weariness.

Some of these feelings could be attitudes of mind rather than emotions – or are they? Whatever the conclusion, all the emotions or
feelings in this group seem to convey a sense of weariness, to have an
air of unconcern about them, almost as though detached, and needing a 'push' to get the person going again!

Although not exactly the same, if we look at each one in this
group, we can see that apathy and listlessness both share inactivity
and lack of interest (the latter is evident in boredom too; languor and
sluggishness are evident in both lethargy and listlessness and there
are other similarities).

Apathy is almost akin to a 'don't care' attitude of mind, perhaps linked with a feeling of inadequacy; however, underlying this can be feelings of hopelessness, disappointment and boredom, and it can even be the result of denied chronic anger (Lindenfield, p.171). Apathy is an emotion which is slow to develop and may often be a result of continually accepting the easy way out:

- you start to buy ready prepared meals increasingly often because you find it takes less effort than preparing meals from scratch – and your husband likes them anyway
- you find that although you like playing tennis, it's easier to watch it on television, and gradually, you don't bother to play at all
- the business you enthusiastically built up has succeeded and you begin to delegate some of the jobs you used to take pride in doing yourself; the business doesn't seem to suffer so you do it more and more, until you don't really *want* to have anything much to do with it. You develop an 'it's OK' attitude and lose the ambitious spark that made you a success. Apathy has begun!

Lethargy is a gradual increase of tiredness and lack of energy and is fairly close to apathy in that it can be linked to a 'can't be bothered' attitude or an 'it's too much for me' feeling. I have put listlessness into this group, as this can develop when we lose interest in life's routine and pleasures and find we lack strength and animation.

CASE STORY

Almost every office worker begins to feel tired towards the end of the afternoon – especially on a Monday! Also, at school or college, students begin to flag at the end of a theoretical session. For these situations, our production staff use rosemary and lemon essential oils as an inhalant (it is best not used on the skin without some training); in a teaching situation, we pass round a tissue from which the students each take a couple of deep breaths; in the office, they love to have a vaporizer going with a few drops of these oils and water in it. In all cases, people perk up almost immediately, and continue with a fresh spurt of energy.

The properties which will help to lift us out of an apathetic or lethargic state are stimulating oils, those which:

- stimulate the digestion
- stimulate the heart
- stimulate the nervous system
- stimulate the mind
- stimulate the blood and/or lymph circulation
- stimulate the respiratory system

– in other words, all oils which have some kind of stimulating property!

Essential Oils

Rosemary *(Rosmarinus officinalis)*
Rosemary is one of the most useful oils for treating emotions (followed closely by peppermint) and apathy is no exception. It is a great tonic to the nervous system; not only that, it is excellent for stimulating a poor blood (and lymphatic) circulation, as well as having a positive effect on a sluggish digestion and a lethargic liver. Add to this its power to stimulate the mind and use of rosemary, with these outstanding stimulating properties, can only spell success for the emotions in this group. Mojay (1996 p.160) recommends it for lack of determination, Keville & Green (1995 p.66) adding that it increases perception and creativity; all of these are necessary attributes in order to help apathy and its fellow emotions.

Peppermint *(Mentha x piperita)*
Peppermint is well-known for its neurotonic properties and its power to stimulate the mind, thus aiding mental fatigue and apathy (Price & Price, 1999 p.333). Anyone who has used peppermint oil for a cold or to unblock their sinuses will know its speedy ability to decongest and clear the head which suggests it will aid mental clarity. Its stimulating properties, which also include stimulation of the digestive system and appetite, suggest it would be effective on all three emotions on this list; this could in part be due to its cell-regenerating properties too. Keville & Green (1995 p.65) suggest that it unblocks emotions which have 'stuck', so if anger is underlying the apathy, as

Lindenfield (1997 p.161) suggests it can, peppermint, as it is well-known to soothe irritation of the skin, may help here to soothe any hidden or 'stuck' anger.

Juniper *(Juniperus communis)*
A well-known cleansing and purifying oil, juniper is also neurotonic, stimulating the nerves, digestive system, liver and appetite into action. These tonic properties suggest that it would be beneficial when one is lethargic, 'detached' or inactive as well as weary and lacking interest in anything. Juniper's combined stimulating actions should strengthen willpower and restore determination.

Ginger *(Zingiber officinale)*
Ginger is a good tonic oil, stimulating and invigorating. While it is successfully tackling fatigue, it can not only lift the spirits, but also, Battaglia (1997 p.167) tells us it sharpens the senses. Its stimulating properties could also be a great help to someone in a debilitated state, helping to get rid of weariness and restore determination to make an effort. Mojay (1996 p.79) suggests that ginger will help someone with a lack of drive, activating the willpower and stimulating initiative, both of which are needed when trying to combat apathy, lethargy and listlessness.

Lemon *(Citrus limon)*
Although lemon is not known for neurotonic properties, it is an immunostimulant, and when one is low in spirits for a long period of time, resistance to simple ailments like coughs and colds, cold sores and tummy upsets is low. Lemon has a long list of attributes to help physical health, including those mentioned above, so for these alone it should be an excellent oil to use for the emotions in this group. Its aroma is refreshing and uplifting, so we would expect it to clear the mind and lift the spirits. Lawless (1994 p.163) suggests it for tiredness and sluggishness, both of which are symptoms of lethargy and listlessness.

Sweet Marjoram *(Origanum majorana)*
Marjoram is a powerful neurotonic (Price & Price 1999 p.337) and is energizing to anyone in a low state. Helpful for debility, it will lift

weariness and stabilize the mind. As it is a respiratory tonic, it will help deepen the breath, which will, in turn, bring more fresh oxygen into the lungs to liven you up. This in itself is energizing indicating its use for chronic lethargy.

Clary Sage *(Salvia sclarea)*

Clary is neurotonic, and so beneficial for the mental fatigue which apathy, lethargy and listlessness seem to portray. It is a detoxifying oil, and helped by its decongestant properties, it may, while ridding the body of toxins, detoxify and decongest the mind also, clearing the head and restoring a feeling of well-being; as Mojay (1996 p.63) aptly puts it, it gives a 'mental-emotional uplift' and restores clarity. It is regenerative, so sad or 'lethargic' cells can benefit from this and renew life from within themselves, throwing off the dead, apathetic, lethargic and listless cells.

Cypress *(Cupressus sempervirens)*

Another neurotonic oil, cypress will revitalize the person who expresses the emotions in this group. The fact that it increases the flow of venous blood, which never flows as easily as arterial blood even in a healthy person, will help increase energy and vigour, as it speeds up the circulation sending fresh oxygenated blood around the body more quickly – and therefore to the brain; this may, as a consequence, give us increased perception, helping us to be optimistic and 'get a move on'! Fischer-Rizzi (1990 p.91) tells us that cypress strengthens the nervous system.

There are other essential oils with properties which stimulate the nervous, digestive and circulatory systems and would be helpful for the emotions in this group:

- basil *(Ocimum basilicum);* nerve and mental stimulant, digestive stimulant (especially the liver)
- coriander *(Coriandrum sativum);* nerve, mental and digestive stimulant
- geranium *(Pelargonium graveolens);* nerve stimulant, digestive stimulant (particularly the liver) and lymph circulation stimulant
- nutmeg *(Myristica fragrans);* nerve, digestive and circulation stimulant (care needed in use)

- rose otto *(Rosa damascena);* nerve stimulant, general and respiratory tonic
- sage *(Salvia officinalis);* nerve, digestive and circulatory tonic (care needed in use).

Mood Swings, Moodiness

Emotional Imbalance, Moodiness, Mood Swings, Temperamental

- moodiness
  gloomy, sulky, crestfallen, miserable, pensive, touchy, irritable, cross, dismal, downcast, pensive, temperamental, touchy, melancholic, inconsistent, variable
- temperamental
  capricious, emotional, erratic, excitable, impatient, irritable, moody, sensitive, touchy, inconsistent, unpredictable
- inconsistent, contradictory, changeable, unstable
- sensitive
  temperamental, touchy, irritable.

Common to three of the above are being touchy and irritable, with inconsistent featuring in the first two and temperamental in the first and last. One does not have to be 'in a mood' to be temperamental – it can be simply a part of one's character. This is not really an emotional group; it is more a reflection of varying emotions delicately intertwined, a question, rather, of emotions being out of balance. A mood lasts much longer than an emotion and is a less intense sensation, sometimes lasting an hour or two and sometimes going on for days (Lindenfield, 1997 p.21).

Zevon & Tellagen (1982) found, by recording and examining people's moods every day, that these fall into two different dimensions, 'positive' and 'negative':

- 'Positive' moods can vary from feeling full of life and enthusiastic to feeling relaxed and tired, but still 'friendly'.
- 'Negative' moods can vary from feeling relaxed to feeling antagonistic and worried.

[The] times when we feel high positive and low negative effect together will be experienced as pleasant. We feel happy or satisfied. By contrast, high negative and low positive effect combine to give us an unpleasant time, when we may feel sorry, or lonely, or simply unhappy.

Wood, 1990

General moodiness can affect us all, male and female, and various things can bring on the changes, whether for good or bad: the weather, work, the children, our health, etc. Most of us (I hope!) spend the majority of our time in a stable, happy mood, but when any of the emotions above 'attack us', essential oils can help lift us out of it. A person who is temperamental by nature – part of his/her personality – needs not only essential oils, but also a good measure of practice in positive thinking, to help the oils in their balancing action.

Mood swings in females, when they are alternately irritable and good-natured, unhappy and happy and generally inconsistent, are more often than not connected to the reproductive system. These moods are usually evident just before each period (forming part of premenstrual syndrome, PMS) and during the menopause.

Several essential oils are balancing, both to the health and to the mind, and hormonal oils are helpful for PMS as well as the menopause, but something else which needs to be considered is the aroma itself. This is a very personal thing – and quite important. It is possible that what will help one person will not help another if the aroma is not liked.

CASE STORY

Marlene was having really bad mood problems at work which were affecting her relationships with the other staff, one of whom suggested she try aromatherapy – she had done a two-day course and told Marlene to buy clary sage, which would 'do the trick'. However, Marlene hated the smell and, needless to say, there was not much improvement in her condition. Then she met a friend who knew a professional aromatherapist. During the subsequent consultation, she made up a blend of oils not including clary sage, but using lavender, marjoram and geranium, which are all both sedative and tonic, making a well-balanced mix. Marlene was advised to use this every night, starting two weeks after her period had finished up to the start of, and during, the next one. Even at the first month, the staff felt Marlene was more like her old self, and after four months, she was a new woman at these times (to her husband's delight as well!). I should add here that the therapist had advised a change in eating and drinking habits too, which obviously played an important part in the eventual results.

In selecting essential oils for mood changes, the main property to consider is one of balance; should the moodiness be due to female hormonal activity, oils which are also oestrogen-like would be the best choice. So we have two properties:

• calming, sedative and neurotonic (therefore balancing)
• oestrogen-like.

Essential oils:

Clary Sage *(Salvia sclarea)*
This is the classic choice for moodiness in connection with PMS or menopausal problems, as it is oestrogen-like in action. However, it can still be chosen by those without these problems, as it is both calming and neurotonic. Its antispasmodic action should help calm any irritable feelings which may be part of the mood experienced, and if there is any jealousy or envy, it will help these as well. It is recommended by Mojay (1996 p.63) for changing moods and emotional confusion.

Cypress *(Cupressus sempervirens)*
This oil, too, is hormone-like, being an ovarian stimulant. It is also neurotonic and both calming and sedative, so is a good choice for those with PMS or difficulties with the menopause. Its antispasmodic and calming properties are indicated for any irritability showing itself. Fischer-Rizzi (1990 p.91) recommends it for uncontrollable crying spells and an overburdened nervous system, Keville & Green (1995 p.53) telling us that it increases emotional stamina.

Marjoram *(Origanum majorana)*
Marjoram is neurotonic, sedative and hormone-like, though the latter property is directed towards regulating an overactive thyroid (this can make one irritable and restless when due to an excess of thyroxine, Wingate & Wingate, p.472). Irritability and restlessness, both connected with a change of mood, should be alleviated by the antispasmodic property which marjoram also possesses. Because it is both sedative and uplifting, it is balancing, a very necessary property for mood changes – it will both strengthen and relax the nerves. Keville & Green (1995 p.61) recommend sweet marjoram for those who are unstable emotionally.

Geranium *(Pelargonium graveolens)*
Geranium calms anxiety and is a tonic to the nerves, making it a suitable oil for general moodiness. Its neurotonic property will be of help to those whose mood takes them into depression, whilst the sedative property will help relieve agitation or irritation, aided also by its antispasmodic and anti-inflammatory properties. Lawless (1990 pp.148–149) gives it as helping melancholy and moodiness.

Lavender *(Lavandula augustifolia)*
Lavender is an excellent oil for general moodiness. Although not hormone-like, it is both calming and sedative and its neurotonic property recommends it for melancholy; being also cardiotonic, it helps strengthen the heart (Price & Price, 1999 pp.329–330). Its anti-inflammatory and antispasmodic properties should be useful for a temperamental person. Lawless (1990 p.161) suggests its usefulness for emotional instability and fluctuating mood states, no doubt because of its balancing properties.

Other oils which could help with moodiness and its associated feelings are:

- mandarin (Citrus reticulata); a strong sedative
- neroli (Citrus aurantium var. amara – flowers); relaxing and tonic
- ylang ylang (Cananga odorata); both tonic and calming; antispasmodic, when irritation is present

- sweet thyme (Thymus vulgaris, alcohol chemotype); neurotonic and cardiotonic. Several authors cite it for mental instability and melancholy.

There are numerous other emotions which will enter our feelings at some stage in our lives and it is not possible to write about every single one, nor is it always possible to state categorically which essential oils will help. I believe that the oils one particularly likes would also be beneficial in many instances. My husband, Len, for example, finds geranium helpful for most of his needs – and it happens to be his favourite oil! If one of the emotions below is linked with any other emotion, look at the oils in all the different emotion detailed above which are relevant to your feelings.

Sources of oil suggestions for the following emotions give the author's name only.

Timidity

> For God did not give us a spirit of timidity, but a spirit of power and of self-discipline.
>
> 2 Timothy 1:7

Timidity, Sensitivity, Shyness, Inadequacy, Unworthiness, Underachievement, Lack of Confidence

My suggestion here is to make your choice from all the essential oils which are stimulating, with those which uplift as a basis. Look for the oils which will stimulate more than one system and use two or three of these. You may even find it helpful to look at the oils which help allay fear.

At the same time, practise self-discipline, with love (directed for this set of emotions towards yourself) and positive thinking. If carried out faithfully, this will, together with the essential oils, achieve a spirit of power and an ability to do what you previously never thought possible. Look out for oils which are:

- neurotonic (to boost and strengthen the nervous system)

- stimulating to the circulatory (including lymph), digestive, respiratory and reproductive systems
- mentally stimulating.

Essential Oils

Basil *(Ocimum basilicum)*
Basil, as well as being a tonic to the nerves, is a mental stimulant and is stimulating to the liver and the digestive system as a whole. The fact that it is also cardiotonic and helpful in the case of over-rapid heartbeat (tachycardia), qualifies its use for emotions in this category. Keville & Green recommend it for lack of self-confidence. According to Battaglia, basil gives mind strength and clarity.

Fennel *(Foeniculum vulgare)*
Known for its hormone-like qualities, fennel has a stimulating effect on the reproductive system, for both menstruation and the production of breast milk. It is a respiratory tonic and also cardiotonic, recommended for palpitations and tachycardia. Fennel has a stimulating effect on the digestive system, stimulating the appetite and also the movement of food through the intestines (helping constipation). Although it is not known to be neurotonic, fennel could still be effective for emotions in the timidity group because of the long list of tonic properties.

Sweet marjoram *(Origanum majorana)*
Sweet marjoram is, in my opinion, one of the most useful essential oils and in cases of timidity and related emotions it is no exception. It is a nerve, respiratory and digestive tonic and is also recommended for palpitations and tachycardia; these last two properties indicate that it could be helpful when fear is part of the emotion. Mojay cites it as an oil to use if you are feeling that no-one cares, and Keville & Green recommend it for loneliness.

Rosemary *(Rosmarinus officinalis)*
Once again, rosemary is in the recommended list – it is a very useful essential oil, both for physical and mental problems. Neurotonic, cardiotonic, stimulating to the digestive and reproductive systems and

reputed to be a sexual tonic, these qualities well qualify it as an aid for this group of emotions. One of its best-known properties is that of a mental stimulant, so it will improve perception and therefore creativity (Keville & Green). Mojay writes that it brings self-determination, confirming that it should be a good choice for poor self-image and lack of self-confidence.

Peppermint *(Mentha x piperita)*
A neurotonic which stimulates the reproductive and digestive systems, peppermint also stimulates the mind. These are all useful properties for emotions in this category.

Other oils which may help this class of emotions are:

- bergamot *(Citrus bergamia);* lack of confidence (Fischer-Rizzi); promotes optimism (Mojay)
- ginger *(Zingiber officinale);* boosts confidence and morale, dispels self-doubt (Mojay); sharpens the senses (Battaglia)
- rose otto *(Rosa damascena);* self-nurturing, self-esteem (Holmes)
- thyme *(Thymus vulgaris);* self-doubt, poor self-confidence, restores morale (Mojay)
- ylang ylang *(Cananga odorata);* lack of self-confidence (Battaglia, Fischer-Rizzi).

Confusion

Confusion, Uncertainty, Perplexity, Bewilderment, Irresoluteness, Indecisiveness

More states of mind than emotional, these are likely to be experienced very often by people who fall into the timidity group and would be experienced mostly in cases where timidity and its related feelings are not a personality trait. I feel that the essential oils above would also be helpful here, especially those which stimulate the mind into action and strengthen it at the same time.

I would like to add the following essential oils specifically recommended for indecision and confusion by other writers:

- basil *(Ocimum basilicum);* indecision (Battaglia)
- clary *(Salvia sclarea);* indecision (Mojay)
- lemon *(Citrus limon);* aids decision-making (Fischer-Rizzi and Keville & Green); disperses confusion (Mojay)
- rosemary *(Rosmarinus officinalis);* dispels confusion (Davis).

Airy-fairy

Airy-fairy, Illogical, Prone to Day-dreaming, Not Grounded, Romantic, Forgetful

This again, with its related traits, is more a state of mind than an emotion. We all like to day-dream; however, some people are occasionally longer in this state than is healthy for them and it could develop into apathy. What I feel is needed here are sedative oils to 'bring you back to earth', but choosing those which are also neurotonic to boost the whole body and mind.

Because the following oils contain linalool, a strong sedative component (Schnaubelt, 1995), they would be a good choice:

- mandarin *(Citrus reticulata);* a strong sedative
- neroli *(Citrus aurantium var. amara,* flowers); sedative, neurotonic
- ylang ylang *(Cananga odorata);* sedative.

Other oils which should help are:

- clary *(Salvia sclarea);* calming to parasympathetic nervous system, neurotonic
- cypress *(Cupressus sempervirens);* calming and neurotonic
- lavender *(Lavandula angustifolia);* calming and neurotonic
- sweet marjoram *(Origanum majorana);* calming and neurotonic.

Keville & Green recommend cedarwood and sandalwood for their grounding effects; Mojay suggests clary and patchouli. Davis also suggests patchouli and Battaglia recommends ginger. Holmes gives clary sage as being helpful for 'scattered thinking', absent-mindedness and unrealistic ideas.

Secretiveness

Reserved, reticent, withdrawn

Secretiveness suggests a controlled 'holding in', as sometimes happens with flatulence. Essential oils which help this often uncomfortable condition and can stimulate the digestive system as a whole (sluggishness) should be useful here. Catarrh is something which needs to be let out too, but is often difficult in chronic cases, which suggests that anticatarrhal oils may also be useful.

I can find nothing in other books referring specifically to this group of emotions, but three essential oils have all required properties; others with one or two of the helpful properties can be found in Chapter 8 in the relevant oil profile:

- ginger (Zingiber officinalis); anticatarrhal, carminative (relieves flatulence), digestive tonic
- peppermint (Mentha x piperita); anticatarrhal, carminative (relieves flatulence), digestive tonic
- rosemary (Rosmarinus officinalis); anticatarrhal, carminative (relieves flatulence), digestive tonic.

Conclusion

We have seen just how many emotions there are which affect life and the way it is lived. Our personalities are shaped not only by the way people react to these emotions, but also by the type of emotions experienced most often. I hope that this chapter shows how, just as our own, individual emotions can shape our personality, the 'personalities' of the essential oils can be used to transform destructive emotions into positive ones.

8 *A-Z of Essential Oils*

Essential Oils

There have been so many books written on aromatherapy which give information about essential oils, such as history and how they are made, that I don't want to use valuable space here going into detail about what are now familiar facts. However, I shall select as many points as are needed which are important and relevant to the understanding of this book.

Essential oils are powerful healing substances which can help us in times of trouble when our physical and mental balance is disturbed (Price, 1991). Although aromatherapy *per se* has been in existence only since the 1930s, aromatic plants have been used since antiquity to cleanse both the body and the mind.

An essential oil is the most concentrated plant extract known and is obtained only by distillation of the specific plant material, apart from citrus fruits, whose 'essential oil' is taken by a cold extraction process known as expression (literally pressing the fruit; if you squeeze the empty skin of a fresh orange into a candle flame, the small 'flashes' it produces are its essential oil). In the process of distillation, the plant material yields its volatile essential oil molecules into the steam, which, as it cools, condense into water with the essential oil floating on the top. The resultant water also contains plant molecules, but only those which are soluble in water – on the whole, mostly those which are not volatile. These distilled waters are also of value medicinally, weaker and generally not requiring dilution.

Valuable medicinal plant components (whether or not they contain essential oil molecules inside their cells) can also be extracted by using solvents of different kinds, although the finished product, like the waters, is not as concentrated as an essential oil:

- Alcohol; one of the most common solvents (used in herbal medicine) is alcohol, in which many plant components are soluble. The plants used for Bach flower remedies originally yielded their constituents also to alcohol, to make the mother tincture from which the remedies are made.
- Vegetable oils; olive or sunflower oil are the usual solvents used to obtain the medicinal properties from plants which have hardly any essential oil, like hypericum (St John's Wort) and calendula. In a process called maceration, the chopped up (macerated) plant material is put into a vegetable oil and left in the sun for several days before being filtered. The resulting oil can be used for application or massage. For extra effects, essential oils can also be added.

There are hundreds of essential oil-bearing plants, not all of them used in aromatherapy; of those which are, we will be looking only at a selection of those which are effective on more than one emotional problem, to ease the choice – and the pocket! There is not space to feature here every essential oil mentioned in the text, even though they may be effective for one or two of the emotional difficulties described; the selected oils are those which feature most often and in the majority of the emotions a person may experience.

Underneath each emotional experience and for each essential oil is a list (in italics) of the physical properties which I believe should help that particular emotion. Only those physical properties applicable to the relevant emotion are given, although each essential oil presented may possess many others. This is for simplification, as these are the specific properties discussed in Chapters 5–7.

In this list of properties, those which are relevant to the essential oil being discussed are in bold, for easy recognition and to evaluate its usefulness quickly. The physical problems which each property can alleviate are also given, as this may be of help in your final selection should any of these ailments be present at the time you are selecting oils for your emotional condition.

Should more than one emotion need help, as in grief, by looking at the additional emotion, you may find essential oils which overlap and therefore fulfil both requirements. In other words, you can 'kill two birds with one stone' (or 'love two birds with one kiss' as one of the participants in my Canadian workshop suggested!).

As the properties of each oil vary, select those which you feel have the most attributes for you; also refer to Chapter 7, as often other emotions may be a part of your personal experience. For example, the properties required to relieve jealousy do not always involve those which relieve anger, but if anger is part of your particular situation, these properties will be needed.

For simplicity, the common name of the essential oil is given first, followed by the botanical name; however, the latter is the name to use – *always* – when purchasing essential oils, as several botanical species have the same common name, and without specifying, you may be given the wrong essential oil. Take marjoram for example; the plant we use in aromatherapy is *Origanum majorana* – 'true' or 'sweet' marjoram – but also available on the aromatherapy market is *Thymus mastichina,* whose common name is marjoram too – 'Spanish' marjoram – although it is a different plant, with different properties.

A–Z

Basil *(Ocimum basilicum)*

> ... we greatly esteem it because it smelleth sweet, and (as some think) comforteth the brain.
>
> John Swan, *Speculum Mundi*

There are many varieties of basil, most of them grown in Mediterranean countries, though it is also grown for its essential oil in Nepal. Some varieties have very small delicate leaves *(Ocimum minimum)*, while others have big, rich-smelling leaves, like *Ocimum basilicum,* the one I like to put in our salads. There are green-leaved basils and dark purple-leaved basils; strong-flavoured basils and weak-flavoured basils; 'exotic' basils and 'sweet' basils. 'Exotic' basils have a high content of estragol (known also as methyl chavicol) – a rather powerful constituent which needs care in use, whereas 'sweet basils' have a low estragol content, making them preferable for use in aromatherapy as they present no risk to the health. John Gerard (1512–1612), author of *Great Herbal* (1597), is supposed to have said that the smell of basil is good for the heart:

it taketh away sorrowfulness, which cometh of melancholy, and maketh a man merry and glad.

In aromatherapy today, basil is valued for these same attributes; it is a tonic to the nerves, making it an excellent choice for depression and fatigue; it is clearing to the head and, as it is also relaxing, it is one of the best oils to balance and regulate the nervous system; it is effective for confused minds and mental strain of any kind.

Cautions
Exotic basil (eugenol and thymol types), available from some suppliers, should not be used during the early months of pregnancy.

Properties
Grief group:
analgesic, balancing, calming, **cardiotonic**, **cicatrizant**, digestive, immunostimulant, **mental stimulant**, **nerve tonic**, sedative

- *analgesic* – relief of pain in migraine, rheumatoid arthritis
- *cardiotonic* – tonic to heart; arrhythmia, arteriosclerosis, tachycardia
- *cicatrizant* (healing) – stomach ulcers
- *mental stimulant* – uplifting to mind
- *neurotonic* – tonic to nerves, convalescence, debility, depression, mental strain

Anger group:
anticatarrhal, **anti-inflammatory**, **antispasmodic**, calming, carminative (relieving flatulence), **cicatrizant**, sedative

- *anti-inflammatory* – reduction of inflammation in gout, rheumatoid arthritis, wasp stings
- *antispasmodic* – relieves gastric spasm and muscle cramp
- *cicatrizant* (healing) – stomach ulcers

Fear group:
antispasmodic, **cardiotonic**, calming, **digestive**, **mental stimulant**, **nerve tonic**, respiratory tonic, sedative

- *antispasmodic* – relieves gastric spasm and muscle cramp
- *cardiotonic* – tonic to heart; arrhythmia, arteriosclerosis, tachycardia
- *mental stimulant* – uplifting to mind
- *digestive tonic* – stimulates liver and digestive secretions, sluggish digestion
- *nervous system regulator* – anxiety, epilepsy, nervous insomnia, general nervousness, travel sickness, vertigo
- *neurotonic* – tonic to nerves; convalescence, debility, depression, mental strain

Jealousy group:
antifungal, **antiviral**, cicatrizant, **detoxifying**, litholytic (breaks down stones)

- *antifungal* – fungus not known
- *antiviral* – viral hepatitis
- *cicatrizant* (healing) – stomach ulcers

Confusion group:
balancing (tonic and sedative), **cardiotonic**, decongestant, **mental stimulant**

- *balancing*
- *cardiotonic* – tonic to heart, arrhythmia, arteriosclerosis, tachycardia
- *mental stimulant*

Timidity group:
cardiotonic, **mental stimulant**, **nerve tonic**, circulation stimulant, respiratory tonic

- *cardiotonic* – tonic to heart, arrhythmia, arteriosclerosis, tachycardia
- *mental stimulant*
- *nervous system regulator* – anxiety, epilepsy, nervous insomnia, general nervousness, travel sickness, vertigo

Airy-fairy group:
astringent, **cardiotonic**, sedative

* *cardiotonic* – tonic to heart; arrhythmia, arteriosclerosis, tachycardia

Secretiveness:
anticatarrhal, **carminative** (relieves flatulence), **digestive tonic**

* *carminative* – relieves flatulence
* *digestive stimulant* – sluggish digestion

Bergamot *(Citrus bergamia)*

Being a citrus fruit, bergamot is not distilled for its oil; the essential oil is in the rind and is easily extracted by expression *(see page 65)*. Italy is the main producer and the fruit is grown by grafting a bergamot branch onto a 'host' orange tree, which gives a healthier crop; in Cyprus you can find one grafted tree on the edge of an orange plantation, for family use; the farmer's wife makes delicious and popular candied peel, often served with afternoon tea.

Bergamot is one of the ingredients in the original and famous eau de Cologne and is also used in the production of Earl Grey tea (I often make my own, by putting one drop of the essential oil on each Assam tea bag – or 10 drops into a quarter of good quality loose tea, shaking well in a tin to allow the oil to permeate throughout – wonderful!).

A tonic as well as a calming oil, bergamot is balancing to the nervous system. It is particularly good for depression, in which the refreshing and uplifting aroma plays an important part. In fact, its physical and psychological effects have been verified during use on patients in a psychiatric clinic to relieve fear as well as calm anxiety (Fischer-Rizzi, 1990 pp.70–72). It is especially beneficial in cases of grief, as so many different emotions which bergamot can relieve surface in this complicated state of mind.

Properties
Grief group:
analgesic, **balancing, calming**, cardiotonic, **cicatrizant, digestive,** immunostimulant, mental stimulant, **neurotonic, sedative**

- *balancing* (sedative and tonic)
- *calming* – insomnia
- *cicatrizant* (healing) – burns
- *neurotonic* – digestive system, central nervous system
- *sedative* – agitation
- *digestive* – loss of appetite.

Anger group:
anticatarrhal, anti-inflammatory, **antispasmodic**, **calming**, carminative (relieving flatulence), **cicatrizant**, **sedative**

- *antispasmodic* – colic, indigestion
- *cicatrizant* (healing) – burns
- *calming* – insomnia
- *sedative* – agitation

Fear group:
antispasmodic, cardiotonic, **calming**, **digestive**, mental stimulant, **nerve tonic**, respiratory tonic, **sedative**

- *antispasmodic* – colic, indigestion
- *calming* – insomnia
- *sedative* – agitation
- *neurotonic* – digestive system, central nervous system
- *stomachic* – loss of appetite

Jealousy group:
antifungal, **antiviral**, **cicatrizant**, detoxifying, litholytic (breaks down stones)

- *antiviral* – herpes simplex 1
- *cicatrizant* (healing) – burns

Chamomile (Roman) *(Chamaemelum nobile)*

> It is profitable for all sorts of agues that come either from phlegm or melancholy *(and)* taketh away weariness *(and)* comforteth both it *(the head)* and the brain.
>
> Culpeper (1616–1654)

The essential oil from Roman chamomile is taken from cultivated plants with double daisy-like flower heads. Grown in various European countries, it has been used for over 2000 years; the Greeks called it 'ground apple' on account of its aroma. In the distillation process it produces azulene, which gives it a pale blue colour and is partly responsible for its healing ability on skin problems. It should not be confused with German chamomile *(Chamomilla recutita)*, which contains much more azulene (giving it a deep blue, almost blue-black colour) and therefore having a stronger action on skin inflammation.

Roman chamomile is one of the most efficient oils for insomnia and for the nervous system generally – especially for children. Chamomile tea, made from the double flower heads, is a popular drink in France – and a favourite of aromatherapists in the UK and America.

A low-growing variety is recommended instead of grass for those people who do not like mowing the lawn; it not only makes a thick carpet eventually, but gives off its clean, refreshing aroma when walked upon.

Properties
Grief group:
analgesic, balancing, **calming**, cardiotonic, **cicatrizant**, **digestive**, immunostimulant, mental stimulant, **nerve tonic**, sedative

- *calming and sedative* – insomnia, irritability, migraine, nervous shock
- *cicatrizant* (healing) – boils, burns, wounds
- *digestive* – indigestion, loss of appetite
- *general health tonic*

Anger group:
anticatarrhal, **anti-inflammatory, antispasmodic, calming,**
carminative, **cicatrizant, sedative**

- *anti-inflammatory* – eczema, gout, inflamed skin, rheumatism,
  urticaria, skin irritation, cracked nipples, inflamed gums, neuritis
- *antispasmodic* – headaches, migraine, neuromuscular tension,
  infantile diarrhoea
- *cicatrizant* (healing) – boils, burns, wounds
- *calming and sedative* – insomnia, irritability, migraine, nervous
  shock
- *carminative* – relieving flatulence

Fear group:
antispasmodic, cardiotonic, **calming, digestive,** mental stimulant,
nerve tonic, respiratory tonic, **sedative**

- *antispasmodic* – headaches, migraine, neuromuscular tension,
  infantile diarrhoea
- *calming and sedative* – insomnia, irritability, migraine, nervous
  shock
- *digestive* – indigestion, loss of appetite

Jealousy group:
antifungal, antiviral, **cicatrizant,** detoxifying, litholytic (breaks down
stones)

- *cicatrizant* (healing) – boils, burns, wounds

Guilt group:
analgesic, cardiotonic, **cicatrizant,** decongestant, detoxifying,
digestive

- *cicatrizant* – boils, burns, wounds
- *digestive tonic* – indigestion, loss of appetite

Secretiveness:
anticatarrhal, **carminative, digestive tonic, sudorific**

- *carminative* – flatulence
- *digestive tonic* – indigestion, loss of appetite
- *sudorific* – encourages sweating

Clary Sage *(Salvia sclarea)*

> Some brewers of Ale and Beere doe put it (the infused plant) into their drinks to make it more heady, fit to please drunkards, who thereby, according to their several dispositions, become either dead drunke, or foolish drunke, or madde drunke.
>
> Lobel

Clary sage is often confused with sage, yet it is a completely different plant; it has huge leaves and flowers and can grow to almost a metre and a half in height. It has the most heady aroma, which not everyone likes; however, it produces a valuable oil for women's problems. 'Salvia' means health and 'sclarea' means clear and I believe it is as good as its word. It is a powerful oil, and immediately after use, one should not drink any alcohol, as it enhances the effect – not good if you have to drive!

Properties
Grief group:
analgesic, balancing, **calming**, cardiotonic, cicatrizant, digestive, immunostimulant, mental stimulant, **nerve tonic**, sedative

- *calming* – to the parasympathetic nervous system
- *neurotonic* – nervous fatigue

Anger group:
anticatarrhal, anti-inflammatory, **antispasmodic**, **calming**, carminative (relieving flatulence), cicatrizant, sedative

- *antispasmodic*
- *calming* – to the parasympathetic nervous system

Fear group:
antispasmodic, cardiotonic, **calming**, digestive, mental stimulant, **nerve tonic**, respiratory tonic, sedative

- *antispasmodic*
- *calming* – to the parasympathetic nervous system
- *neurotonic* – nervous fatigue

Jealousy group:
antifungal, antiviral, cicatrizant, **detoxifying**, litholytic (breaks down stones)

- *antifungal* – dermal fungal infections
- *detoxifying*

Guilt group:
analgesic, cardiotonic, cicatrizant, **decongestant**, **detoxifying**, digestive

- *decongestant* – painful and difficult menstruation
- *detoxifying*

Mood swings:
balancing (calming and tonic), **hormone-like**

- *balancing* – to nervous system
- *hormone-like* – PMS, menopause, hot flushes

Cypress *(Cupressus sempervirens)*

Traditionally found in graveyards, the cypress is a pretty tree, tall and slim, having light foliage and attractive round, almost smooth cones. The cypress (also known as Italian cypress), grown for its essential oil, is found mainly in southern Europe and has been described as 'an exclamation mark on a happy landscape' (Valnet, 1980). The wood is hard, but easy to work and was used by the Phoenicians to build ships and houses (Price, Price-Parr 1996). All parts of the tree are used to extract the essential oil (twigs together with leaves and cones), which has a light woody aroma. Its best-known attributes are its astringent and styptic properties – reducing production of body fluids, such as perspiration, sebum and blood, the latter being where it has its most important effect. Its next most important property, and useful for the emotions, is its tonic effect on the nervous system.

Incidentally, if you meet someone who talks too much (verbal diarrhoea), (see Case Story p.12) try giving him or her cypress oil on a tissue; the fruits have been used traditionally for diarrhoea:

> The cones or nuts ... are good to stop fluxes of all kinds, as spitting of blood, diarrhoea, dysentry, the immoderate fluxes of the menses, involuntary miction; they prevent bleeding of the gums and fasten loose teeth.
>
> Culpeper's Complete Herbal p.110

Properties
Grief group:
analgesic, **balancing**, **calming**, cardiotonic, cicatrizant, digestive, immunostimulant, mental stimulant, **nerve tonic**, sedative

- *balancing* (calming and neurotonic)
- *calming* – irritability, regulates sympathetic nervous system
- *neurotonic* – debility

Anger group:
anticatarrhal, anti-inflammatory, **antispasmodic**, **calming**, carminative (relieving flatulence), cicatrizant, sedative

- *antispasmodic* – cramp
- *calming* – irritability, regulates sympathetic nervous system

Fear group:
antispasmodic, cardiotonic, **calming**, digestive, mental stimulant, **nerve tonic**, respiratory tonic, sedative

- *antispasmodic* – cramp
- *calming* – irritability, regulates sympathetic nervous system
- *neurotonic* – debility

Mood swings:
balancing, hormone-like

- *balancing* (calming and neurotonic)
- *hormone-like* – ovary problems

Frankincense *(Boswellia carteri)*

This small tree has grown wild in the Red Sea area and north-east Africa since biblical times. It was once considered as precious as gold, which is why it was one of the gifts brought to Jesus by the Wise Men; in fact, it is mentioned about 20 times in the Bible, mostly in the Old Testament, as the Jews used it in their religious rites.

Frankincense (sometimes referred to as olibanum) is a gum extracted from the frankincense bush by cutting into the bark; to protect itself from this wound, it produces a whitish, milky liquid, which, on exposure to the air, eventually hardens to a yellowy-brown gum. The gum is then distilled to give the essential oil, which has a rich, yet fresh, balsamic aroma. The gum is produced mainly in Iran and Lebanon.

I believe that it is because the tree is wounded and immediately begins to heal itself that the essential oil is one of the best for renewing human damaged cell tissue and therefore for healing emotional wounds especially grief. Culpeper is reputed to have given it as a great nerve strengthener (thus good for depression) and as an aid to the memory, though not mentioned in his *Complete Herbal*.

Properties
Grief group:
analgesic, balancing, calming, cardiotonic, **cicatrizant**, digestive, **immunostimulant**, mental stimulant, **nerve tonic**, sedative

- *analgesic* – rheumatism, sports injuries
- *cicatrizant* – scars (including stretch marks), ulcers, wounds
- *immunostimulant* – weak immune system
- *nerve tonic* – nervous depression

Anger group:
anticatarrhal, **anti-inflammatory**, antispasmodic, calming, carminative (relieving flatulence), **cicatrizant**, sedative

* *anticatarrhal* – asthma, bronchitis
* *anti-inflammatory* – rheumatism
* *cicatrizant* – scars (including stretch marks), ulcers, wounds

Fear group:
antispasmodic, cardiotonic, calming, digestive, mental stimulant, **nerve tonic**, respiratory tonic, sedative

* *nerve tonic* – nervous depression

Jealousy group:
antifungal, antiviral, **cicatrizant**, detoxifying, litholytic (breaks down stones)

* *cicatrizant* – scars (including stretch marks), ulcers, wounds

Guilt group:
analgesic, cardiotonic, **cicatrizant**, decongestant, detoxifying, digestive

* *analgesic* – rheumatism, sports injuries
* *cicatrizant* – scars (including stretch marks), ulcers, wounds

Apathy group:
circulation and/or lymph stimulant, digestive tonic, mental stimulant, **nerve tonic**, nervous system regulator, respiratory tonic

* *nerve tonic* – nervous depression

Timidity group:
cardiotonic, mental stimulant, **nerve tonic**, circulation stimulant, respiratory tonic

* *nerve tonic* – nervous depression

Geranium *(Pelargonium graveolens)*

Originally a native of Africa, geranium was brought to Europe in the late 17th century. Geraniums are grown commercially in France, Egypt, Morocco, China and the island of Réunion, the best oil for aromatherapy considered to be that from Réunion island, although geranium oils from China (slightly different in composition – and less expensive) are also frequently used. There are many species of geranium, the one from which the essential oil is obtained having small, highly aromatic and slightly hairy leaves with 'lacy' edges; the flowers are delicate and usually pink and unscented. It was thought in medieval times to be protective:

> Snakes will not go
> where geraniums grow.
>
> cited in Lawless, 1994 p.149

Geranium is a balancing oil, able to relieve stress as well as alleviating depression and uplifting the mind.

Properties
Grief group:
analgesic, **balancing**, **calming**, cardiotonic, **cicatrizant**, digestive, immunostimulant, mental stimulant, **nerve tonic**, sedative

- *analgesic* – facial neuralgia, osteoarthritis, rheumatism
- *balancing* – calming and stimulating
- *calming* – anxiety, agitation
- *cicatrizant* – burns, cuts, ulcers, uterine haemorrhage, stretch marks, wounds
- *nerve tonic* – debility, nervous fatigue

Anger group:
anticatarrhal, **anti-inflammatory**, **antispasmodic**, calming, carminative (relieving flatulence), cicatrizant, sedative

- *anti-inflammatory* – arthritis, colitis, pruritis, rheumatism, tonsillitis

- *antispasmodic* – colic, cramp, gastroenteritis, painful menstruation

Fear group:
antispasmodic, cardiotonic, **calming**, digestive, mental stimulant, **nerve tonic**, respiratory tonic, sedative

- *antispasmodic* – colic, cramp, gastroenteritis, painful menstruation
- *calming* – anxiety, agitation
- *nerve tonic* – debility, nervous fatigue

Jealousy group:
antifungal, antiviral, **cicatrizant**, detoxifying, litholytic (breaks down stones)

- *antifungal* – athlete's foot and other skin and nail fungi, *Candida albicans*
- *cicatrizant* – burns, cuts, ulcers, uterine haemorrhage, stretch marks, wounds

Guilt group:
analgesic, cardiotonic, **cicatrizant**, **decongestant**, detoxifying, digestive

- *analgesic* – facial neuralgia, osteoarthritis, rheumatism
- *cicatrizant* – burns, cuts, ulcers, uterine haemorrhage, stretch marks, wounds
- *decongestant* – breast congestion, lymph congestion

Apathy group:
circulation and/or lymph stimulant, digestive tonic, mental stimulant, **nerve tonic**, nervous system regulator, respiratory tonic

- *nerve tonic* – debility, nervous fatigue

Mood swings:
balancing, hormone-like

- *balancing* – calming and stimulating

Confusion group:
balancing (tonic and sedative), cardiotonic, **decongestant**, mental stimulant

- *balancing* – calming and stimulating
- *decongestant* – breast congestion, lymph congestion

Timidity group:
cardiotonic, mental stimulant, **nerve tonic**, circulation stimulant, respiratory tonic

- *nerve tonic* – debility, nervous fatigue

Ginger *(Zingiber officinalis)*

Ginger is native to eastern Asia, and is cultivated extensively in Nigeria, the West Indies, China and Jamaica. The essential oil, which does not contain the 'hotness' reminiscent of ginger, is taken from the rhizome (root). The Chinese have used ginger root for centuries as a herbal remedy against many ailments.

Its principal action is on the digestive tract, though it also has other properties which indicate its usefulness for some emotional conditions.

Properties
Grief group:
analgesic, balancing, calming, cardiotonic, cicatrizant, **digestive**, immunostimulant, mental stimulant, **nerve tonic**, sedative

- *analgesic* – angina, painful indigestion, rheumatism, toothache
- *digestive stimulant* – constipation, loss of appetite, sluggish digestion, nausea
- *general tonic* – fatigue

Anger group:
anticatarrhal, anti-inflammatory, antispasmodic, calming, **carminative**, cicatrizant, sedative

- *anticatarrhal* – chronic bronchitis

- *carminative* – flatulence

Fear group:
antispasmodic, cardiotonic, calming, **digestive stimulant**, mental
stimulant, nerve **tonic**, respiratory tonic, sedative

- *digestive stimulant* – constipation, loss of appetite, sluggish
  digestion, nausea
- *general tonic* – fatigue

Guilt group:
analgesic, cardiotonic, cicatrizant, decongestant, detoxifying,
digestive stimulant

- *analgesic* – angina, painful indigestion, rheumatism, toothache
- *digestive stimulant* – constipation, loss of appetite, sluggish
  digestion, nausea

Timidity group:
cardiotonic, mental stimulant, nerve **tonic**, circulation stimulant,
respiratory **tonic**

- *general tonic* – nervous fatigue

Apathy group:
circulation and/or lymph stimulant, **digestive stimulant**,
mental stimulant, nerve **tonic**, nervous system regulator, respiratory
tonic

- *digestive stimulant* – constipation, loss of appetite, sluggish
  digestion, nausea
- *general tonic* – fatigue

Secretiveness:
anticatarrhal, carminative, digestive stimulant

- *anticatarrhal* – chronic bronchitis
- *carminative* – flatulence

- *digestive stimulant* – constipation, loss of appetite, sluggish digestion, nausea

Juniper *(Juniperus communis)*

> The berries … strengthen the brain, fortify the sight, by strengthening the nerves are good for the agues, help the gout and sciatica, and strengthen the limbs of the body.
>
> Culpeper's *Complete Herbal* p.205

Juniper is an evergreen shrub grown all over the Mediterranean. The berries are distilled to obtain juniper berry oil, which is more expensive and has slightly different properties from the oil obtained by distilling branches with both needles and berries. The latter is the one usually available on general sale, juniper berry oil being used mainly to flavour gin.

Juniper oil is stimulant to the kidneys and an excellent antiseptic (especially valuable in cases of cystitis) as well as being antitoxic and purifying.

> The cleansing properties of juniper work on the mental/emotional plane as well as the physical. It is a psychically purifying oil … Juniper seems to clear 'waste' from the mind just as it does from the body.
>
> Davis 1991, pp.191–2

Caution
Juniper oil should not be used when kidneys are inflamed or diseased, in case of overstimulating them.

Properties
Grief group:
analgesic, balancing, calming, cardiotonic, cicatrizant, **digestive**, immunostimulant, mental stimulant, **nerve tonic**, sedative

- *analgesic* – arthritis, muscular aches and pains, rheumatism
- *digestive tonic* – cirrhosis, loss of appetite
- *nerve tonic* – debility, fatigue

Anger group:
anticatarrhal, anti-inflammatory, antispasmodic, calming, carminative (relieving flatulence), cicatrizant, sedative

* *anticatarrhal* – bronchitis, rhinitis
* *anti-inflammatory*

Fear group:
antispasmodic, cardiotonic, calming, **digestive tonic**, mental stimulant, **nerve tonic**, respiratory tonic, sedative

* *digestive tonic* – cirrhosis, loss of appetite
* *nerve tonic* – debility, fatigue

Jealousy group:
antifungal, antiviral, cicatrizant, **detoxifying**, **litholytic**

* *detoxifying* – skin problems, kidneys, digestive system
* *litholytic* – bladder and kidney stones

Guilt group:
analgesic, cardiotonic, cicatrizant, decongestant, **detoxifying, digestive tonic**

* *analgesic* – arthritis, muscular aches and pains, rheumatism
* *detoxifying* – skin problems, kidneys, digestive system
* *digestive tonic* – cirrhosis, loss of appetite

Apathy group:
circulation and/or lymph stimulant, **digestive tonic**, mental stimulant, **nerve tonic**, nervous system regulator, respiratory tonic

* *digestive tonic* – cirrhosis, loss of appetite
* *neurotonic* – debility, fatigue

Timidity group:
cardiotonic, mental stimulant, **nerve tonic**, circulation stimulant, respiratory tonic

- *nerve tonic* – debility, fatigue

Secretiveness:
anticatarrhal, carminative (relieves flatulence), **digestive tonic**

- *anticatarrhal* – bronchitis, rhinitis
- *digestive tonic* – cirrhosis, loss of appetite

Lavender *(Lavandula angustifolia)*

> Two spoonfuls of the distilled water of the flowers *(of spike lavender)* help them that have lost their voice, the tremblings and passions of the heart, and faintings and swoonings, applied to the temples or nostrils, to be smelt unto.
>
> Culpeper's *Complete Herbal* p.210

Whenever I use lavender I think of the superb Provençal mountainsides, with rows of mostly blue, but very occasionally pink and white, lavender flowers gently swaying in the breeze and filling the air with their aroma. French lavender is the best in the world, especially wild-picked, though wild lavender essential oil rarely sees a bottle, due to the expense of collecting it.

The beautiful purple flowers dominating the lower landscape are not lavender at all, as most people think, but lavandin *(Lavandula* x *intermedia)*, a cross between true lavender and spike lavender *(Lavandula spica*, a much bigger plant), which produces more essential oil and has a more camphoraceous aroma. I tell you this because some commercial oils sold in the shops as lavender are in reality, lavandin, so if it is lavender you want, always check that its Latin name is on the bottle – *Lavandula angustifolia*. Lavandin is a useful oil too, but you need to know which one you are buying.

Lavender grows at an altitude of more than 500 metres (1650 feet), which is why it is often missed by tourists – lavandin grows well below this height. The oil is distilled from the first 20–25 cm (8–10 in) of the flowering tops.

Lavender has many useful properties, its most famous being its healing effect on burns. It is great for headaches too, especially if you can catch it as soon as you feel it coming on. This popular essential oil is in most aromatherapy skin care products as it is balancing, which means that it will benefit both dry and greasy skins, helping them to return to normal. Law (1982), an authority on botanic medicine, says that 'the plant signifies love and long life'.

Properties
Grief group:
analgesic, balancing, calming, cardiotonic, cicatrizant, digestive, immunostimulant, mental stimulant, **nerve tonic,** sedative

- *analgesic* – arthritis, muscular aches and pains, rheumatism
- *balancing* – both calming and uplifting, nervous system regulator
- *cardiotonic* – tachycardia (rapid heartbeat)
- *cicatrizant* – burns, scabs, scars, varicose ulcers, wounds
- *nerve tonic* – debility, melancholy

Anger group:
anticatarrhal, **anti-inflammatory, antispasmodic, calming,** carminative (relieving flatulence), **cicatrizant, sedative**

- *anti-inflammatory* – eczema, insect bites, phlebitis, sinusitis, otitis (inflammation of the ear), cystitis, bruises, sprains, acne, herpes, pruritis (itching)
- *antispasmodic* – cramp, spasmodic coughing
- *calming, sedative* – headaches, migraine, insomnia, sleep problems, anxiety
- *cicatrizant* – burns, scabs, scars, varicose ulcers, wounds

Fear group:
antispasmodic, cardiotonic, calming, digestive, mental stimulant, **nerve tonic,** respiratory tonic, **sedative**

- *antispasmodic* – cramp, spasmodic coughing
- *cardiotonic* – tachycardia (rapid heartbeat)
- *calming, sedative* – headaches, migraine, insomnia, sleep problems, anxiety
- *nerve tonic* – debility, melancholy

Jealousy group:
antifungal, antiviral, **cicatrizant**, detoxifying, litholytic (breaks down stones)

* *antifungal* – candida, athlete's foot (including infection of the nails)
* *cicatrizant* – burns, scabs, scars, varicose ulcers, wounds

Guilt group:
analgesic, **cardiotonic**, **cicatrizant**, decongestant, detoxifying, digestive

* *analgesic* – arthritis, muscular aches and pains, rheumatism
* *cardiotonic* – tachycardia (rapid heartbeat)
* *cicatrizant* – burns, scabs, scars, varicose ulcers, wounds

Apathy group:
circulation and/or lymph stimulant, digestive tonic, mental stimulant, **nerve tonic**, **nervous system regulator**, respiratory tonic

* *nerve tonic* – debility, melancholy
* *nervous system regulator*

Mood swings:
balancing, hormone-like

* *balancing* – both calming and uplifting, nervous system regulator

Confusion group:
balancing (tonic and sedative), **cardiotonic**, decongestant, mental stimulant

* *balancing* – both calming and uplifting, nervous system regulator
* *cardiotonic* – tachycardia (rapid heartbeat)

Timidity group:
cardiotonic, mental stimulant, **nerve tonic**, circulation stimulant, respiratory tonic

- *cardiotonic* – tachycardia (rapid heartbeat)
- *nerve tonic* – debility, melancholy

Airy-fairy group:
astringent, **cardiotonic, sedative**

- *cardiotonic* – tachycardia (rapid heartbeat)
- *calming, sedative* – headaches, migraine, insomnia, sleep problems, anxiety

Lemon *(Citrus limon)*

Lemon and other citrus fruit essential oils are not obtained by distillation but by expression – a 'cold' method of extraction. The essential oil is in the rind, which is pressed to express the oil. Sometimes, and especially with orange, the whole fruit is pressed; the essential oil floats on top of the juice and is separated off. The principal area of lemon production is Sicily, although it is cultivated extensively in other Mediterranean countries, especially Spain. Here, I have collected wild and garden lemons as big as grapefruit, though the smaller varieties are usually cultivated for their fruit. As the oil is so near to the exterior, it is best to buy oil from organic fruits which have not been sprayed with pesticides, or waxed.

Because expressed oils contain components other than volatile ones, for example, natural waxes, they do not have the same keeping qualities and the waxes may separate out – this does not impair the effects of the oil.

The fresh smell of lemon is cleansing and uplifting to the mind, increasing concentration; indeed, research in Japan on typing errors showed that there were 54 per cent fewer mistakes in those who were exposed to a lemon aroma (Fischer-Rizzi, 1990 p.120). However, it is mainly a calming oil, possessing almost sedative qualities.

Properties
Grief group:
analgesic, balancing, **calming**, cardiotonic, cicatrizant,
digestive, immunostimulant, mental stimulant, nerve tonic,
sedative

- *calming and sedative* – headaches, insomnia, nightmares
- *digestive* – gastritis, nausea, painful digestion, loss of appetite, stomach ulcers
- *immunostimulant* – white cell deficiency
- *mental stimulant* – increases concentration

Anger group:
anticatarrhal, **anti-inflammatory**, **antispasmodic**, **calming**, **carminative**, cicatrizant, sedative

- *anti-inflammatory* – boils, gout, insect bites, rheumatism
- *antispasmodic* – diarrhoea
- *calming* – headaches, insomnia, nightmares
- *carminative* – flatulence

Fear group:
antispasmodic, cardiotonic, **calming**, **digestive**, **mental stimulant**, nerve tonic, respiratory tonic, sedative

- *antispasmodic* – diarrhoea
- *calming* – headaches, insomnia, nightmares
- *digestive* – gastritis, nausea, painful digestion, loss of appetite, stomach ulcers
- *mental stimulant* – increases concentration

Jealousy group:
antifungal, **antiviral**, cicatrizant, detoxifying, litholytic (breaks down stones)

- *antifungal* – thrush
- *antiviral* – colds, herpes, veruccas, warts

Guilt group:
analgesic, cardiotonic, cicatrizant, decongestant, detoxifying, **digestive**

- *digestive* – gastritis, nausea, painful digestion, loss of appetite, stomach ulcers

Apathy group:
circulation and/or **lymph stimulant, digestive tonic, mental
stimulant**, nerve tonic, nervous system regulator, respiratory tonic

- *circulatory* – hypertension, phlebitis, poor circulation, thrombosis,
  varicose veins
- *digestive* – gastritis, nausea, painful digestion, loss of appetite,
  stomach ulcers
- *mental stimulant* – increases concentration

Confusion group:
balancing (tonic and sedative), cardiotonic, decongestant, **mental
stimulant**

- *mental stimulant* – increases concentration

Timidity group:
cardiotonic, **mental stimulant**, nerve tonic, **circulation
stimulant**, respiratory tonic

- *mental stimulant* – increases concentration
- *circulation stimulant* – hypertension, phlebitis, poor circulation,
  thrombosis, varicose veins

Airy-fairy group:
astringent, cardiotonic, **sedative**

- *sedative/ calming* – headaches, insomnia, nightmares

Secretiveness:
anticatarrhal, **carminative, digestive tonic**

- *carminative* – flatulence
- *digestive tonic* – gastritis, nausea, painful digestion, loss of
  appetite, stomach ulcers

Marjoram *(Origanum majorana)*

> Our Common Sweet Marjoram is warming and comforting in
> cold diseases of the head ... taken inwardly or outwardly
> applied. The decoction thereof being drunk, helps ... old
> griefs of the womb.
>
> Culpeper's *Complete Herbal* p.227

A native of Europe and central Asia, marjoram yields a sweet-smelling
essential oil, unlike Spanish marjoram *(Thymus mastichina)*, often sold
– wrongly – as the aromatherapist's marjoram and having a sharper
aroma. The leaves are a soft shade of grey-green and are covered with
down-like hairs, which, as in all plants in the Labiate family, protect
the tiny essential oil glands on the outside of the leaves.

Marjoram has been used for centuries as a culinary herb (especially with sausages), its success in this field probably being due to its
digestive properties (Mabey, 1988). It is the most sedative of all
essential oils, and as it also has neurotonic properties, it is balancing
too.

The ancient Egyptians used sweet marjoram for healing and over-
coming grief and it is known today for its calming and comforting
effect on the mind. The name of the plant is derived from the Greek
and means 'joy of the mountain', and the plant itself is a symbol of
happiness. The Greeks used to plant it on graves, convinced that it
would help their loved ones to sleep in peace and happiness
(Clarkson, 1972 p.130); this bears out the Egyptian connection as a
comforter in grief.

Properties
Grief group:
analgesic, **balancing**, **calming**, cardiotonic, cicatrizant, **digestive
tonic**, immunostimulant, mental stimulant, **nerve tonic**, sedative

- *analgesic* – arthritis, migraine, muscular pain, rheumatism,
  toothache
- *balancing*
- *calming* – agitation, anxiety, epilepsy, insomnia, migraine,
  psychoses, sexual obsessions, vertigo

- *digestive tonic* – indigestion, gastro-duodenal ulcers
- *nerve tonic* – debility, mental instability, anguish, nervous depression

Anger group:
anticatarrhal, anti-inflammatory, **antispasmodic**, **calming**, **carminative**, cicatrizant, sedative

- *antispasmodic* – colic, muscular spasm, respiratory spasm, nervous spasm
- *calming* – agitation, anxiety, epilepsy, insomnia, migraine, psychoses, sexual obsessions, vertigo
- *carminative* – relieves flatulence

Fear group:
antispasmodic, cardiotonic, **calming**, **digestive tonic**, mental stimulant, **nerve tonic**, **respiratory tonic**, sedative

- *antispasmodic* – colic, muscle spasm, respiratory spasm, nervous spasm
- *calming* – agitation, anxiety, epilepsy, insomnia, migraine, psychoses, sexual obsessions, vertigo
- *digestive tonic* – indigestion, gastro-duodenal ulcers
- *nerve tonic* – debility, mental instability, anguish, nervous depression
- *respiratory tonic* – nervous breathing

Guilt group:
analgesic, cardiotonic, cicatrizant, decongestant, detoxifying, **digestive tonic**

- *analgesic* – arthritis, migraine, muscular pain, rheumatism, toothache
- *digestive tonic* – indigestion, gastro-duodenal ulcers

Apathy group:
circulation and/or lymph stimulant, **digestive tonic**, mental stimulant, **nerve tonic**, nervous system regulator, **respiratory tonic**

- *digestive tonic* – indigestion, gastro-duodenal ulcers
- *nerve tonic* – debility, mental instability, anguish, nervous depression
- *respiratory tonic* – nervous breathing

Mood swings:
balancing, hormone-like

- *balancing* – both calming and tonic
- *hormone-like* – hyperthyroidism

Confusion group:
balancing (tonic and sedative), cardiotonic, decongestant, mental stimulant

- *balancing* – calming and neurotonic

Timidity group:
cardiotonic, mental stimulant, **nerve tonic**, circulation stimulant, **respiratory tonic**

- *nerve tonic* – debility, mental instability, anguish, nervous depression
- *respiratory tonic* – nervous breathing

Airy-fairy group:
astringent, cardiotonic, **calming/sedative**

- *calming/sedative* – agitation, anxiety, epilepsy, insomnia, migraine, psychoses, sexual obsessions, vertigo

Secretiveness:
anticatarrhal, **carminative**, **digestive tonic**

- *carminative* – flatulence
- *digestive* – indigestion, gastro-duodenal ulcers

Melissa *(Melissa officinalis)*

> The later age, together with the Arabians and Mauritanians, affirme Balme to be singular good for the heart, and to be a remedie against the infirmities thereof; for Avicen in his booke written of the infirmities of the heart, teacheth that Bawme makes the heart merry and joyfull, and strengtheneth the vital spirits.
>
> Gerard, 1545–1612

Originating in southern Europe, but quite common in Britain, melissa is a small perennial herb with a wonderful aroma – indeed, its local name is 'heart's delight'.

Unfortunately, the essential oil glands are very delicate, and as there is not much oil in the leaves anyway, much can be lost on the way to the distillery simply by the weight of plant on plant; it cannot be harvested if it is damp, or with dew on it. All these parameters make it a very expensive essential oil, but in my view it is worth every penny! When we bought our first 250 ml of melissa, eight years ago, only one litre had been distilled in the whole of the south of France; most of the plant production was – and still is – used in the making of melissa tea. Now, melissa is grown by many more farmers and 60 litres were distilled this year.

It is often referred to as the 'elixir of life', and people who have drunk melissa tea every day have been found to have lived longer, healthier lives. Recent research has shown the efficacy of melissa's sedative properties on vegetative dystonia and its symptoms of excitability, headaches, palpitations and restlessness.

> An essence of Balm, given in Canary wine every morning, will renew youth, strengthen the brain, relieve languishing nature and prevent baldness.
>
> *London Dispensary,* 1696

Properties
Grief group:
analgesic, balancing, **calming**, cardiotonic, cicatrizant, **digestive tonic**, immunostimulant, mental stimulant, nerve tonic, **sedative**

- *calming* – hysteria, palpitations, headaches, vertigo, over-excitability
- *digestive tonic* – indigestion, nausea, morning sickness, sluggish liver
- *sedative* – to central nervous system

Anger group:
anticatarrhal, **anti-inflammatory**, **antispasmodic**, **calming**, carminative (relieving flatulence), cicatrizant, **sedative**

- *anti-inflammatory* – bee stings
- *antispasmodic* – stomach cramp
- *calming* – hysteria, palpitations, headaches, vertigo, over-excitability
- *sedative* – insomnia, calming to central nervous system

Fear group:
antispasmodic, cardiotonic, **calming**, **digestive tonic**, mental stimulant, nerve tonic, respiratory tonic, **sedative**

- *antispasmodic* – stomach cramp
- *calming* – hysteria, palpitations, headaches, vertigo, over-excitability
- *digestive tonic* – indigestion, nausea, morning sickness, sluggish liver
- *sedative* – insomnia, calming to central nervous system

Jealousy group:
antifungal, antiviral, cicatrizant, detoxifying, litholytic (breaks down stones)

- *antiviral* – *Herpes simplex 1*

Guilt group:
analgesic, cardiotonic, cicatrizant, decongestant, detoxifying, **digestive tonic**

- *digestive tonic* – indigestion, nausea, morning sickness, sluggish liver

Apathy group:
circulation and/or lymph stimulant, **digestive tonic**, mental
stimulant, nerve tonic, nervous system regulator, respiratory tonic

- *digestive tonic* – indigestion, nausea, morning sickness, sluggish
  liver

Airy-fairy group:
astringent, **calming/sedative**, cardiotonic

- *calming* – hysteria, palpitations, headaches, vertigo, over-excitability
- *sedative* – insomnia, calming to central nervous system

Secretiveness:
anticatarrhal, carminative (relieves flatulence), **digestive tonic**

- *digestive tonic* – indigestion, nausea, morning sickness, sluggish liver

Niaouli *(Melaleuca viridiflora)*

Occasionally called gomenol, niaouli originated from New Caledonia,
from the region of Gomene. It is distilled from the leaves of the tree,
which grows to around 15 metres in height and is from the same
family as cajeput and tea tree.

Much of the niaouli oil available is reconstituted and smells almost
exclusively of eucalyptol (the main component in eucalyptus) so be
sure to buy from a reliable source. The first impression of the aroma
of genuine niaouli is a bit like eucalyptol also, but this is soon followed by a multiplicity of aromas, including orange blossom, bitter
almond, vanilla and banana. It is still a medicinal-smelling essential
oil and is a must for the medicine chest!

It is a respiratory and vaginal cleanser and is effective – to a lesser
extent – on the circulation (Collin 1997).

Properties
Grief group:
analgesic, balancing, calming, cardiotonic, cicatrizant, **digestive
tonic**, **immunostimulant**, mental stimulant, **nerve tonic**, sedative

- *analgesic* – labour in childbirth
- *digestive tonic* – gastritis, gastric and duodenal ulcers, diarrhoea
- *immunostimulant* – activates body's defences, augments white cells and antibodies
- *nerve tonic* – post-viral nervous depression

Anger group:
anticatarrhal, anti-inflammatory, antispasmodic, calming, carminative (relieves flatulence), cicatrizant, sedative

- *anticatarrhal* – bronchitis, coughs, colds, chronic catarrh
- *anti-inflammatory* – sinusitis, rhinopharyngitis, bronchitis, blepharitis (inflammation of the eyelids), vulvovaginitis, urethritis, prostatitis, inflammation of the coronary arteries

Fear group:
antispasmodic, cardiotonic, calming, **digestive tonic**, mental stimulant, **nerve tonic**, respiratory tonic, sedative

- *digestive tonic* – gastritis, gastric and duodenal ulcers, diarrhoea
- *nerve tonic* – post-viral nervous depression

Jealousy group:
antifungal, **antiviral**, cicatrizant, detoxifying, **litholytic** (breaks down stones)

- *antiviral* – viral hepatitis, viral enteritis, genital herpes
- *litholytic* – gallstones

Guilt group:
analgesic, cardiotonic, cicatrizant, decongestant, detoxifying, **digestive tonic**

- *analgesic* – labour in childbirth
- *digestive tonic* – gastritis, gastric and duodenal ulcers, diarrhoea

Apathy group:
circulation and/or **lymph stimulant, digestive tonic,**

mental stimulant, nerve tonic, nervous system regulator, respiratory tonic

- *circulation and/or lymph stimulant* – varicose veins, haemorrhoids
- *digestive tonic* – gastritis, gastric and duodenal ulcers, diarrhoea

Mood swings:
balancing, **hormone-like**

- *hormone-like* – irregular periods, lack of periods, scanty periods

Timidity group:
cardiotonic, **circulation stimulant**, mental stimulant, **nerve tonic**, respiratory tonic

- *circulation stimulant* – varicose veins, haemorrhoids
- *nerve tonic* – post-viral nervous depression

Secretiveness:
anticatarrhal, carminative (relieves flatulence), **digestive tonic**

- *anticatarrhal* – bronchitis, coughs, colds, chronic catarrh
- *digestive tonic* – gastritis, gastric and duodenal ulcers, diarrhoea

Peppermint *(Mentha* x *piperita)*

Surprisingly enough, although most oils used in aromatherapy need the heat of the sun to produce first-class oils, peppermint prefers lots of daylight; a product of northern temperate climates, it doesn't thrive so well in the south of France. The best oils are produced from plants grown in cooler countries; in fact, the plant used for the oil originated in Mitcham in England. Mitcham plants have been exported all over the world, identified as 'Mitcham (pepper)mint'.

The peppermint plant had widespread use in the East thousands of years ago, principally as a tonic. It was cultivated in Egypt – a valued herb, used as a tithe, in which respect it is mentioned twice in the New Testament when Jesus was addressing the Pharisees:

Woe to you Pharisees, because you give God a tenth of your mint, rue and all other kinds of garden herbs, but you neglect justice and the love of God. You should have practised the latter without leaving the former undone.

Luke, 11:42

The aroma is easily recognized. Whole, non-rectified peppermint oil has an additional 'sweetness' compared to the menthol smell extracted from peppermint oils for toothpaste, ice cream, digestive tablets, chewing gum, etc.; hundreds of tons of the oil are produced every year to keep up with the demand by the food and pharmaceutical industries.

Be careful if you plant peppermint in your garden as it soon takes over! Our peppermint is everywhere, as we hardly ever have time to weed the garden. However, we do use several stems at a time regularly in salads and I add it to our tea too. One drop of peppermint oil in a pot of weak tea (and drunk without milk) is a good analgesic – and better for your stomach than aspirin.

Caution

Because of its strong aroma, the recommended dilution should be observed; in warm vapour inhalations, two drops maximum should be used and the eyes should be covered. It should never be used on babies on account of its strong aroma.

Properties

Grief group:

analgesic, balancing, calming, cardiotonic, cicatrizant, **digestive tonic**, immunostimulant, **mental stimulant**, **nerve tonic**, sedative

- *analgesic* – headaches, migraine, neuralgia, sciatica
- *digestive tonic* – indigestion, nausea, painful digestion, digestive problems, irritable bowel syndrome
- *mental stimulant* – aids memory
- *nerve tonic* – apathy, nervous vomiting, travel sickness, palpitations, vertigo

Anger group:
anticatarrhal, anti-inflammatory, antispasmodic, calming, **carminative,** cicatrizant, sedative, **soothing**

- *anticatarrhal* – bronchial asthma, bronchitis
- *anti-inflammatory* – bronchitis, colitis, cystitis, eczema, enteritis, gastritis, hepatitis, laryngitis, sinusitis
- *antispasmodic* – colic, gastric spasm
- *carminative* – flatulence
- *soothing* – skin irritation, rashes, redness, nettle rash, hives

Fear group:
antispasmodic, cardiotonic, calming, **digestive tonic, mental stimulant, nerve tonic,** respiratory tonic, sedative

- *antispasmodic* – colic, gastric spasm
- *digestive tonic* – indigestion, nausea, painful digestion, digestive problems, irritable bowel syndrome
- *mental stimulant* – aids memory
- *nerve tonic* – apathy, nervous vomiting, travel sickness, palpitations, vertigo

Jealousy group:
antifungal, antiviral, cicatrizant, detoxifying, litholytic (breaks down stones)

- *antifungal* – ringworm, skin fungal infections
- *antiviral* – herpes, viral hepatitis

Guilt group:
analgesic, cardiotonic, cicatrizant, **decongestant,** detoxifying, **digestive tonic**

- *analgesic* – headaches, migraine, neuralgia, sciatica
- *decongestant* – cirrhosis
- *digestive tonic* – indigestion, nausea, painful digestion, digestive problems, irritable bowel syndrome

Apathy group:
circulation and/or lymph stimulant, **digestive tonic, mental stimulant, nerve tonic,** nervous system regulator, respiratory tonic

- *digestive tonic* – indigestion, nausea, painful digestion, digestive problems, irritable bowel syndrome
- *mental stimulant* – aids memory
- *nerve tonic* – apathy, nervous vomiting, travel sickness, palpitations, vertigo

Confusion group:
balancing (tonic and sedative), cardiotonic, **decongestant, mental stimulant**

- *decongestant* – cirrhosis
- *mental stimulant* – aids memory

Timidity group:
cardiotonic, **mental stimulant, nerve tonic,** circulation stimulant, respiratory tonic

- *mental stimulant* – aids memory
- *nerve tonic* – apathy, nervous vomiting, travel sickness, palpitations, vertigo

Secretiveness:
anticatarrhal, carminative, digestive tonic

- *anticatarrhal* – bronchial asthma, bronchitis
- *carminative* – flatulence
- *digestive tonic* – indigestion, nausea, painful digestion, digestive problems, irritable bowel syndrome

Pine *(Pinus sylvestris)*

Also known as Scots Pine, this hardy tree can be found growing all over Europe and is indigenous in the colder regions of Russia and

Scandinavia. The twigs, with needles and cones, are distilled to obtain the essential oil, which has a fresh, antiseptic aroma. Cones from one of the pine species growing in Norway can be used to dye wool different shades of orange-yellows.

Pine essential oil is principally antiseptic, especially in purifying the air to keep it free from unwanted bacteria. It also has many other physical properties which are relevant to its use for the emotions – its neurotonic properties in particular.

Properties
Grief group:
analgesic, balancing, calming, cardiotonic, cicatrizant, digestive tonic, immunostimulant, mental stimulant, **nerve tonic**, sedative

- *analgesic* – arthritis, rheumatism, gastralgia, intestinal pains
- *nerve tonic* – debility, fatigue, multiple sclerosis

Anger group:
anticatarrhal, anti-inflammatory, antispasmodic, calming, carminative (relieving flatulence), cicatrizant, sedative

- *anticatarrhal* – respiratory tract, coughs

Fear group:
antispasmodic, cardiotonic, calming, digestive tonic, mental stimulant, **nerve tonic**, respiratory tonic, sedative

- *nerve tonic* – debility, fatigue, multiple sclerosis

Jealousy group:
antifungal, antiviral, cicatrizant, **detoxifying**, **litholytic** (breaks down stones)

- *antifungal* – Candida albicans
- *detoxifying* – purifying
- *litholytic* – gallstones

Guilt group:
analgesic, cardiotonic, cicatrizant, **decongestant, detoxifying,**
digestive tonic

- *analgesic* – arthritis, rheumatism, gastralgia, intestinal pains
- *decongestant* – congested lymph, uterine or ovarian congestion,
  breaks down bronchial secretions
- *detoxifying* – purifying

Apathy group:
circulation and/or lymph stimulant, digestive tonic, mental
stimulant, **nerve tonic**, nervous system regulator, respiratory tonic

- *nerve tonic* – debility, fatigue, multiple sclerosis

Confusion group:
balancing (tonic and sedative), cardiotonic, **decongestant**, mental
stimulant

- *decongestant* – congested lymph, uterine or ovarian congestion,
  breaks down bronchial secretions

Timidity group:
cardiotonic, mental stimulant, **nerve tonic**, circulation stimulant,
respiratory tonic

- *nerve tonic* – debility, fatigue, multiple sclerosis

Secretiveness:
anticatarrhal, carminative (relieves flatulence), digestive tonic

- *anticatarrhal* – respiratory tract, coughs

Rose otto *(Rosa damascena)*

> Sugar of roses is a very good cordial to strengthen the heart
> and spirit ... The syrup of roses ... comforteth the heart and
> resisteth putrefaction and infection ... Red rose water is well

known, it is cooling, cordial, refreshing, quickening the weak and faint spirits.

Culpeper; excerpts from Grieve, 1998 p.691

Two kinds of rose oil are available on the aromatherapy market – rose absolute (which is not a distilled oil, but obtained by solvent extraction) and rose otto, obtained by distillation and, in my opinion, the only one to be used for therapeutic aromatherapy.

Bulgarian roses are reputed to give the best distilled rose oil; like melissa leaves, there is very little oil in the petals (only these are used). The oil is really a by-product of distillation, floating on top of the highly aromatic and precious rose water, the production of which is often the principal aim of the distillers.

Rose is probably capable of more effects than its known properties give it credit for; this may be due to its remarkable aroma, which seems to relax and/or uplift the mind. Rose oil's effect on the spiritual aspect of the human psyche is best expressed by Madame Maury, the lady who introduced aromatherapy to England:

... the rose procures us one thing above all: a feeling of well-being, even of happiness, and the individual under its influence will develop an amiable tolerance.

Maury, 1989

Properties
Grief group:
analgesic, **balancing**, **calming**, cardiotonic, **cicatrizant**, digestive tonic, immunostimulant, mental stimulant, **nerve tonic**, sedative

* *balancing*
* *calming* – emotional shock
* *cicatrizant* – mouth ulcers, skin problems, sprains, wounds
* *nerve tonic* – debility, depression

Anger group:
anticatarrhal, **anti-inflammatory**, antispasmodic, **calming**, carminative (relieving flatulence), **cicatrizant**, sedative

- *anti-inflammatory* – blotchy skin, gingivitis
- *calming* – emotional shock
- *cicatrizant* – mouth ulcers, skin problems, sprains, wounds

Fear group:
antispasmodic, cardiotonic, **calming**, digestive tonic, mental stimulant, **nerve tonic**, respiratory tonic, sedative

- *calming* – emotional shock
- *nerve tonic* – debility, depression

Jealousy group:
antifungal, antiviral, **cicatrizant**, detoxifying, litholytic (breaks down stones)

- *cicatrizant* – mouth ulcers, skin problems, sprains, wounds

Guilt group:
analgesic, cardiotonic, **cicatrizant**, decongestant, detoxifying, digestive tonic

- *cicatrizant* – mouth ulcers, skin problems, sprains, wounds

Apathy group:
circulation and/or lymph stimulant, digestive tonic, mental stimulant, **nerve tonic**, nervous system regulator, respiratory tonic

- *nerve tonic* – debility, depression

Mood swings:
balancing, hormone-like

- *balancing*

Timidity group:
Cardiotonic, mental stimulant, **nerve tonic**, circulation stimulant, respiratory tonic

- *nerve tonic* – debility, depression

Rosemary *(Rosmarinus officinalis)*

> Speaking of rosemary, it overtoppeth all the flowers in the garden, boasting man's rule. It helpeth the brain, strengtheneth the memorie, and is very medicinal for the head. Another property of the rosemary is, it affects the heart. Let this rosmarinus, this flower of men, ensigne your wisdom, love and loyaltie, be carried not only in your hands but in your hearts and heads.
>
> Roger Hackett, 1607

I cannot walk past a rosemary bush without taking my fingers up a stem and smelling them – the aroma is fantastic! We have several rosemary bushes outside our house in France, but haven't tried distilling any yet. Garden legend has it that 'where rosemary thrives, the mistress is master' – oh dear! – we have just planted eight bushes in our garden here in England!

> As for Rosmarine, I lett it run alle over my garden walls, not onlie because the bees love it, but because 'tis the herb sacred to remembrance, and thereto to friendship; whence a sprig of it hath a dumb language that maketh it the chosen emblem at our funeral wakes, and in our buriall grounds.
>
> Sir Thomas More; cited in *Clair,* 1961

The best rosemary for essential oils grows in Spain and Tunisia, though an excellent one also grows in the very southernmost part of Provence. Whenever we are in Spain, we walk in the hills, looking for rosemary bushes to smell – and to take a sprig back to our flat for cooking. Have you ever tried adding a sprig of rosemary to apples when you stew them? The flavour is wonderful! By the way, you do need to wrap it in a small piece of muslin (a bit from a wide bandage will do if you don't have a little spice bag for your bouquet garni).

Rosemary is a versatile oil, helpful for many physical and emotional problems. In the past, it played many roles in the everyday life of England, when, among its uses, it symbolized remembrance, love and loyalty (Grieve, 1998 p.681) at both weddings and funerals and was used to cure headache and heartache (Clarkson, 1972 p.117). It is an excellent stimulant, to the body as well as the mind, waking you up when you are tired but have a lot to do, and lifting the spirits when you are feeling depressed. It is most helpful as a mental stimulant at exam times, as it quickens the memory. 'There's rosemary, that's for remembrance' *(Hamlet)*. Good luck for your next exam!

As a result of its impressive properties, rosemary is indispensable for emotional problems, helping all primary and secondary emotions in more respects than most other oils; the only property it lacks is the ability to calm!

Properties
Grief group:
analgesic, balancing, calming, **cardiotonic**, **cicatrizant**, **digestive tonic**, immunostimulant, **mental stimulant**, **nerve tonic**, sedative

- *analgesic* – migraine, painful digestion
- *cardiotonic* – palpitations, weak heart
- *cicatrizant* – burns, wounds
- *digestive tonic* – indigestion, sluggish digestion, colitis, constipation, painful digestion
- *mental stimulant* – lack of concentration, memory loss, poor memory
- *nerve tonic* – fainting, general debility, general fatigue, hysteria, vertigo

Anger group:
anticatarrhal, **anti-inflammatory**, **antispasmodic**, calming, **carminative**, **cicatrizant**, sedative

- *anticatarrhal* – chronic bronchitis, sinusitis
- *anti-inflammatory* – cystitis, gout, muscular inflammation, earache, rheumatism, inflamed gall bladder
- *antispasmodic* – muscle cramp
- *carminative* – flatulence
- *cicatrizant* – burns, wounds

Fear group:
antispasmodic, **cardiotonic**, calming, **digestive tonic**, **mental stimulant**, **nerve tonic**, respiratory tonic, sedative

- *antispasmodic* – muscle cramp
- *cardiotonic* – palpitations, weak heart
- *digestive tonic* – indigestion, sluggish digestion, colitis, constipation, painful digestion
- *mental stimulant* – lack of concentration, memory loss, poor memory
- *nerve tonic* – fainting, general debility, general fatigue, hysteria, vertigo

Jealousy group:
antifungal, antiviral, cicatrizant, detoxifying, litholytic (breaks down stones)

- *antifungal* – Candida albicans
- *antiviral*
- *cicatrizant* – burns, wounds
- *detoxifying* – hepatitis, jaundice, cirrhosis, enlarged liver, gall-bladder malfunction
- *litholytic* – gallstones

Guilt group:
analgesic, cardiotonic, cicatrizant, decongestant, detoxifying, digestive tonic

- *analgesic* – migraine, painful digestion
- *cardiotonic* – palpitations, weak heart
- *cicatrizant* – burns, wounds
- *decongestant* – headaches, migraine, arteriosclerosis
- *detoxifying* – hepatitis, jaundice, cirrhosis, enlarged liver, gall-bladder malfunction
- *digestive tonic* – indigestion, sluggish digestion, colitis, constipation, painful digestion

Apathy group:
circulation and/or **lymph stimulant, digestive tonic, mental stimulant, nerve tonic**, nervous system regulator, respiratory tonic

- *circulation stimulant* – poor circulation
- *digestive tonic* – indigestion, sluggish digestion, colitis, constipation, painful digestion
- *mental stimulant* – lack of concentration, memory loss, poor memory
- *nerve tonic* – fainting, general debility, general fatigue, hysteria, vertigo

Confusion group:
balancing (tonic and sedative), **cardiotonic, decongestant, mental stimulant**

- *cardiotonic* – palpitations, weak heart
- *decongestant* – headaches, migraine, arteriosclerosis
- *mental stimulant* – lack of concentration, memory loss, poor memory

Timidity group:
cardiotonic, circulation stimulant, mental stimulant, nerve tonic, respiratory tonic

- *cardiotonic* – palpitations, weak heart
- *circulation stimulant* – poor circulation
- *mental stimulant* – lack of concentration, memory loss, poor memory
- *nerve tonic* – fainting, general debility, general fatigue, hysteria, vertigo

Airy-fairy group:
astringent, **cardiotonic**, sedative

- *cardiotonic* – palpitations, weak heart

Secretiveness:
anticatarrhal, carminative, digestive tonic

- *anticatarrhal* – chronic bronchitis, sinusitis
- *carminative* – flatulence

- *digestive tonic* – indigestion, sluggish digestion, colitis, constipation, painful digestion

Sage *(Salvia officinalis)*

> Sage is singularly good for the head and brain, it quickeneth the senses and memory.
>
> Gerard, 1545–1612

> He that would live for aye
> Must eat sage in May.
>
> Medieval saying cited in Grieve, 1998 p.701

The generic name of sage comes from the Latin *salvere*, 'to save' or 'to heal', no doubt because it has been valued for its healing powers for centuries, its medicinal prowess as a sacred herb dating from well before Jesus was born. The species name 'officinalis' denotes that this species (out of over 700) was the 'official' sage of the apothecary's shop at the time Linnaeus named the plant in the mid-18th century.

Sage is indigenous to the countries bordering the Mediterranean; both Spain and France are important countries of production. The harvested plant material is often left to dry before distilling, as it is usually ready at the same time as lavender and lavandin, which have to be distilled more or less straightaway.

> Sage makes a good tea; it helps to prepare the uterus for labour if drunk daily, commencing about three weeks before expected childbirth – and because it is hormone-like, it helps reduce hot flushes prevalent during the menopause.
>
> Bourret, 1981

> It is very profitable for all manner of pains in the head coming of cold or rheumatic humours: as also for all pains of the joints, whether inwardly or outwardly, and therefore helps falling-sickness, the lethargy, lowness of spirits, and the palsy; it is also useful in defluxions of rheum in the head, and for diseases of the chest or breast.
>
> Culpeper: p.311

Caution

As sage may be an emmenagogue (it can induce or regularize menstruation), it is best not used in the first five months of pregnancy; it also dries up breast milk, so, although useful to take away unwanted milk, do not use while breastfeeding if your milk supply is normal. However, it does facilitate delivery *(see above)*.

Properties

Grief group:
analgesic, balancing, calming, cardiotonic, **cicatrizant**, **digestive tonic**, immunostimulant, mental stimulant, **nerve tonic**, sedative

- *analgesic* – angina, rheumatism, toothache
- *cicatrizant* – general healing properties
- *digestive tonic* – indigestion, loss of appetite, sluggish digestion
- *nerve tonic* – alopecia, general debility, nervous debility, tremors, vertigo

Anger group:
anticatarrhal, anti-inflammatory, **antispasmodic**, calming, carminative (relieves flatulence), **cicatrizant**, sedative

- *anticatarrhal* – asthma, bronchitis, coughs, sinusitis
- *antispasmodic* – dysmenorrhoea (painful or difficult menstruation)
- *cicatrizant* – general healing properties

Fear group:
antispasmodic, cardiotonic, calming, **digestive tonic**, mental stimulant, **nerve tonic**, respiratory tonic, sedative

- *antispasmodic* – dysmenorrhoea (painful or difficult menstruation)
- *digestive tonic* – indigestion, loss of appetite, sluggish digestion
- *nerve tonic* – alopecia, general debility, nervous debility, tremors, vertigo

Jealousy group:
antifungal, **antiviral**, **cicatrizant**, detoxifying, litholytic (breaks down stones)

- *antifungal* – Candida albicans
- *antiviral* – genital herpes, thrush, viral enteritis, viral meningitis, viral neuritis
- *cicatrizant* – general healing properties

Guilt group:
analgesic, cardiotonic, **cicatrizant**, **decongestant**, detoxifying, **digestive tonic**

- *analgesic* – angina, rheumatism, toothache
- *cicatrizant* – general healing properties
- *decongestant* – congested lymph
- *digestive tonic* – indigestion, loss of appetite, sluggish digestion

Apathy group:
circulation and/or **lymph stimulant**, **digestive tonic**, mental stimulant, **nerve tonic**, nervous system regulator, respiratory tonic

- *circulation and/or lymph stimulant* – poor circulation, congested lymph
- *digestive tonic* – indigestion, loss of appetite, sluggish digestion
- *nerve tonic* – alopecia, general debility, nervous debility, tremors, vertigo

Mood swings:
balancing, **hormone-like**

- *hormone-like* – conducive to conception, facilitates delivery, menopause, premenopause, sterility

Confusion group:
balancing (tonic and sedative), cardiotonic, **decongestant**, mental stimulant

- *decongestant* – congested lymph

Timidity group:
cardiotonic, **circulation stimulant**, mental stimulant, **nerve tonic**, respiratory tonic

- *circulation stimulant* – poor circulation, congested lymph
- *nerve tonic* – alopecia, general debility, nervous debility, tremors, vertigo

Airy-fairy group:
astringent (reducing secretions), cardiotonic, sedative

- *astringent* – excessive hand or armpit sweating, night sweats

Secretiveness:
anticatarrhal, carminative (relieves flatulence), **digestive tonic**

- *anticatarrhal* – chronic bronchitis, sinusitis
- *digestive tonic* – indigestion, loss of appetite, sluggish digestion

Thyme (sweet) *(Thymus vulgaris* ct *geraniol* and *linalool)*

> The affection of bees for thyme is well known and the fine flavour of the honey of mount Hymettus near Athens was said to be ... of such especial flavour and sweetness that in the minds and writings of the Ancients, sweetness and thyme were indissolubly united.
>
> Grieve, 1998 p.809

Thyme is a small plant which is very easy to grow. It has many varieties, several of which gardeners will be familiar with, but for essential oil of thyme, a tiny-leaved dark-green variety, which forms a bushy, ground-covering shrub, is used. It is grown extensively in the south of France.

There are many chemotypes of *Thymus vulgaris*, two of which are too powerful to be used without knowledge (these are often referred to as 'red' or 'white' thymes), because one of their principal components is a phenol. There are other chemotypes (referred to as 'sweet' thymes because their principal component is an alcohol), with a much gentler action, which makes them more user-friendly.

If thyme is grown from seed, it is referred to as 'population' thyme, as it contains a rich variety of components, including both phenols and alcohols. When a plant is analysed and found to contain predominantly one or the other of these, cuttings (clones) are taken from each so that a whole field of phenol thymes or a whole field of alcohol thymes can be grown. Most thyme oil available is phenolic containing carvacrol or thymol, and to be sure of getting what you want when buying the sweet one, the chemotype must be specified – linalool or geraniol.

One of the advantages of sweet thyme is that it can be used with safety – especially on children; it has a long list of useful indications, many of which are effective on the emotions.

Properties
Grief group:
analgesic, balancing, calming, **cardiotonic**, cicatrizant, digestive tonic, **immunostimulant**, mental stimulant, **nerve tonic**, sedative

- *cardiotonic* – tired heart
- *immunostimulant* – stimulates the production of white cells
- *nerve tonic* – fatigue, nervous insomnia

Anger group:
anticatarrhal, **anti-inflammatory**, **antispasmodic**, calming, carminative (relieves flatulence), cicatrizant, sedative

- *anti-inflammatory* – bronchitis, cystitis, muscular rheumatism, earache, urethritis, vaginitis, eczema, psoriasis
- *antispasmodic* – bronchiole spasm

Fear group:
antispasmodic, cardiotonic, calming, digestive tonic, mental stimulant, **nerve tonic**, respiratory tonic, sedative

- *antispasmodic* – bronchiole spasm
- *nerve tonic* – fatigue, nervous insomnia

Jealousy group:
antifungal, **antiviral**, cicatrizant, detoxifying, litholytic (breaks down stones)

- *antifungal* – Candida albicans
- *antiviral* – verrucae, viral enteritis, repetitive viral attacks

Guilt group:
analgesic, **cardiotonic**, cicatrizant, decongestant, detoxifying, digestive

- *cardiotonic* – tired heart

Apathy group:
circulation and/or lymph stimulant, digestive tonic, mental stimulant, **nerve tonic**, nervous system regulator, respiratory tonic

- *nerve tonic* – fatigue, nervous insomnia

Confusion group:
balancing (tonic and sedative), **cardiotonic**, decongestant, mental stimulant

- *cardiotonic* – tired heart

Timidity group:
cardiotonic, mental stimulant, **nerve tonic**, circulation stimulant, respiratory tonic

- *cardiotonic* – tired heart
- *nerve tonic* – fatigue, nervous insomnia

Airy-fairy group:
astringent, **cardiotonic**, sedative

- *cardiotonic* – tired heart

Ylang ylang *(Cananga odorata)*

Ylang ylang – the name means 'flower of flowers' – is obtained by distilling the beautiful yellow flowers which hang down from the branches. When they first form they are green and hairy and in approximately 20 days they are deep yellow. The finest plants are grown in Madagascar and Réunion Island. The tree blossoms all the year round, but the flowers contain the most – and best – oil during the month of May; they are picked before 10 a.m. to be sure of a good yield.

There are many different qualities available, as the distilling time is long – so the oil can be taken off at various periods along the way. The best oils for the perfume industry are those taken in the early part of distillation; however, I prefer a complete oil for a holistic treatment like aromatherapy, as all the components are then present in the oil, even if the aroma is not quite as exotic.

Although not a prominent oil for the emotions, it does have some good effects (including the reduction of high blood pressure), possibly because it is a balancing oil. When more research is done on it, more useful properties may be discovered.

Properties
Grief group:
analgesic, **balancing**, **calming**, cardiotonic, cicatrizant, digestive tonic, immunostimulant, mental stimulant, nerve tonic, **scalp tonic**, sedative

- *balancing* – calming and tonic
- *calming* – hyperventilation, insomnia, tachycardia
- *scalp tonic* – stimulates hair growth

Anger group:
anticatarrhal, anti-inflammatory, **antispasmodic**, **calming**, carminative (relieves flatulence), cicatrizant, sedative

- *antispasmodic*
- *calming* – hyperventilation, insomnia, tachycardia

Fear group:
antispasmodic, cardiotonic, **calming**, digestive tonic, mental stimulant, nerve tonic, respiratory tonic, sedative

- *antispasmodic*
- *calming* – hyperventilation, insomnia, tachycardia

Apathy group:
circulation and/or lymph stimulant, digestive tonic, mental stimulant, nerve tonic, **scalp tonic**, nervous system regulator, respiratory tonic

- *scalp tonic* – stimulates hair growth

Mood swings:
balancing, hormone-like

- *balancing* – calming and tonic

Confusion group:
balancing (tonic and sedative), cardiotonic, decongestant, mental stimulant

- *balancing* – calming and tonic

Timidity group:
cardiotonic, mental stimulant, nerve tonic, **scalp tonic**, circulation stimulant, respiratory tonic

- *scalp tonic* – stimulates hair growth, tonic to scalp

Carrier oils

Carrier oils are the oils to which essential oils are added to dilute them. For massage, it is important to use a carrier oil which will also benefit the problem being treated; use only therapeutic, not culinary quality in order to obtain more effective results, i.e. oils which have been cold-pressed or macerated.

Cold-pressing

The best vegetable oils (from fruits or seeds) are pressed either in a hydraulic press or, in the case of hard seeds, in a gigantic screw device called an expeller (Price, Price & Smith, 2000 p.7). The resulting oil is called a cold-pressed oil, as very little heat is entailed.

The remaining pulp is sent either to farms as cattle food, or to factories which will extract a further quantity of oil, using very high temperatures and sometimes solvents, resulting in a lower grade oil. These oils, although classed as suitable for food, are not suitable for aromatherapy – especially when treating the emotions; *always* use a cold-pressed oil for aromatherapy.

Maceration

This process is used on plants containing very little essential oil, which would make the price of a distilled oil very expensive. For maceration, the chopped-up plants are put into a basic carrier oil, usually olive or sunflower, and left for several days in the sun; during this time, all the components from the chosen plant which are soluble in vegetable oil are taken up by the base oil. The result is a more beneficial carrier oil – into which can also be added essential oils to benefit the problem further.

As far as the emotions are concerned, macerated oils seem to have the best effects because they always contain some of the volatile properties of the plants from which they are made. I have selected only those oils which could be particularly beneficial to emotional problems requiring self-application or massage.

Almond (sweet) *(Prunus amygdalis var. dulcis)*, cold-pressed

> The oil newly pressed out of Sweet Almonds is a mitigator of pain and all manner of aches.
>
> Gerard, 1545–1612

This is one of the most popular oils for massage, though unfortunately, most people buy the refined oil because the cold-pressed one is more expensive. It is always worth a little extra to have quality! The sweet almond tree is mentioned in the Bible as one of the best fruits in the land of Canaan and there are many other biblical references to it (Grieve, 1998 p.22). Almonds were popular in England in the reign of Elizabeth I, when they were used in cookery as well as for health problems. The oil is beneficial to the skin, soothing the irritation of problems such as eczema and psoriasis.

Calendula *(Calendula officinalis)*, macerated

> Conserve made of the floures and sugar, taken in the morning
> fasting, cureth the trembling of the heart.
>
> Gerard, 1512–1612

The common name of this plant is marigold (from the Virgin Mary
and the glorious, cheerful, golden-orange colour of the flowers); to
save confusion with the African marigold, the first part of the Latin
name is now used as the common name. Calendula has been used for
healing since ancient times by herbalists and has many health properties.

Many people regard it as a weed as it self-seeds itself profusely. I
like it in my garden (we have a field of it in France near the house)
and use the petals sprinkled on salads or made into a tea. According
to Grieve (1998 p.518), an infusion of the flowers was used to treat
fevers, as it promotes perspiration, and she writes that it is in
demand for children's ailments.

Lime blossom *(Tilea cordata)*, macerated

> Lime flowers are ... used in infusion or made into a distilled
> water as household remedies in indigestion, or hysteria, ner-
> vous vomiting or palpitation.
>
> Grieve, 1998 p.486

There are two lime (linden) trees outside our house in France and I
frequently make lime blossom tea if we are there when the tree is in
flower. The lime tree must be fly repellent as, although the bees are
busy on the flowers (except between midday and two o'clock!), we
never get flies in the rooms where the trees are near the house; we *do*
get flies at the back of the house where there are no lime trees, so we
are planting one there next year.

There is a large industry in France in tea from lime blossoms
(*tisane de tilleul* – *tilleul* is French for lime tree), which is most relaxing, and if drunk before going to bed, encourages sleep; the other
industry is the making of the macerated oil.

Melissa *(Melissa officinalis)*, macerated

> Balm is sovereign for the brain, strengthening the memory and powerfully chasing away melancholy.
>
> John Evelyn 1620–1706, a founder of the Royal Society

Also available as a macerated oil is melissa, and if the properties of melissa are taken into account, it is a valuable carrier oil. It possesses calming, sedative and digestive properties, so if it is used for emotions requiring these attributes, it would be of additional benefit. Another advantage is that macerated oil of melissa is much less expensive!

St John's Wort *(Hypericum perforatum)*, macerated

> A tincture of the flowers in spirit of wine is commended against melancholy and madness.
>
> Culpeper (1616–1654)

Andrew Chevallier, giving a case history during a lecture on St John's Wort (hypericum), said that a herb which can deal with physical problems can also deal with an emotional state – in this case depression. Conversely, a plant used for mild depression, in this case, St John's Wort, may also ease some of the underlying physical complaints. This suggests that hypericum would be a beneficial oil to carry essential oils into the body when self-application or massage is used. Like some essential oils, hypericum can ease and strengthen the body by supporting systems that are out of balance (Burrough 1999).

> The virtue of it is thus, if it be put in a man's house, then shall come no wicked spirit therein.
>
> Anthony Ascham or Askham – the name has two possible spellings

Sunflower *(Helianthus annuus)*

Sunflowers, which can grow to an enormous height in a very short time, remind me of the drawing of the sun on sundials (*helios* is

Greek for sun). Each seed head of these gigantic flowers can yield a quarter of a kilogram of seeds, from which the oil is taken. The cold-pressed oil can be difficult to find, but is well worth the effort if you want the therapeutic benefits (not present in the refined oil).

Sunflower oil is beneficial for skin problems and bruises (Price, Price and Smith 2000 p.139) and is helpful for acne and oily conditions of the skin (Reynolds 1993).

Tamanu *(Calophyllum inophyllum)*, cold-pressed

> Tamanu grows mainly in tropical south-east Asia and Polynesia. It has naturalized to Hawaii and is grown in Madagascar also.
>
> Price, Price & Smith 2000 p.143

It makes a beautiful ornamental tree on account of its glossy green leaves – in fact, calophyllum is Greek for 'beautiful leaf'. The cold-pressed oil is a rich dark colour, so if you receive a pale-coloured tamanu, it will be refined and no good for aromatherapy.

It is traditionally used in the South Pacific for its pain-relieving, anti-inflammatory and healing properties; it is also reputed to be an immunostimulant (Schnaubelt, 1993).

Properties
Below are the properties of carrier oils which would benefit the primary emotions; for a full reference of the problems they will benefit, see table 8.1.

Grief group:
analgesic, balancing, calming, cardiotonic, cicatrizant, digestive tonic, immunostimulant, mental stimulant, nerve tonic, sedative

- *calendula* (macerated) – anti-inflammatory, cicatrizant
- *lime blossom* (macerated) – analgesic, calming
- *St John's wort* – cicatrizant
- *sunflower* – cicatrizant
- *tamanu* – analgesic, cicatrizant, immunostimulant

Properties and Indications of Principal Fixed Oils (Carrier Oils)

Refer to main text for details

T = traditional use
X = external use
I = internal use

Oil	Analgesic	Antiinflammatory	Antiirritant, antipruritic	Antispasm	Antiviral	Asthma	Astringent	Burns	Chapped, cracked skin	Cicatrisant, (healing)	Dry skin, scalp	Eczema, dermatitis	Emollient	Haemorrhoids	Psoriasis	Sprains/bruises	Skin toning	Sunburn	Ulcers	Varicose, broken veins	Wounds, sores	Wrinkles, ageing skin	Anxiety, stress	Neuralgia
						Skin and Hair																	**Other**	
Almond sweet / Prunus amygdalis var. dulcis			X								X	X	X		X			X						
Calendula / Calendula officinalis (macerated)		TX		TI			T	T	X	TIX		X				TX			T	TX	TX			
Lime blossom, linden / Tilia europaea, T. cordata (macerated)	X												X									X	TIX	
Melissa / Melissa officinalis (macerated)		X	X	X	X																			
St. John's Wort / Hypericum perforatum (macerated)		X			I			X		T		X	X	X	X	TX	X	X	TX		TX		TI	X
Sunflower / Helianthus annuus													X	X	X	X			X					
Tamanu / Calophyllum inophyllum	TX	TX						T	X	T					X									X

Anger group:
anticatarrhal, anti-inflammatory, antispasmodic, calming, carminative (relieves flatulence), cicatrizant, sedative

- *almond* – anti-inflammatory
- *calendula* (macerated) – anti-inflammatory, antispasmodic, cicatrizant
- *lime blossom* (macerated) – calming
- *St John's wort* – anti-inflammatory, cicatrizant
- *sunflower* – cicatrizant
- *tamanu* – anti-inflammatory, cicatrizant

Fear group:
antispasmodic, cardiotonic, calming, digestive tonic, mental stimulant, nerve tonic, respiratory tonic, sedative

- *calendula* (macerated) – antispasmodic
- *lime blossom* (macerated) – calming

Jealousy group:
antifungal, antiviral, cicatrizant, detoxifying, litholytic (breaks down stones)

- *calendula* (macerated) – cicatrizant
- *St John's wort* – cicatrizant
- *sunflower* – antiviral, cicatrizant
- *tamanu* – cicatrizant

Guilt group:
analgesic, cardiotonic, cicatrizant, decongestant, detoxifying, digestive

- *calendula* (macerated) – cicatrizant
- *lime blossom* (macerated) – analgesic
- *St John's Wort* – cicatrizant
- *sunflower* – cicatrizant
- *tamanu* – cicatrizant

Conclusion

When helping someone with essential oils for any problems – emotional or physical – it is essential to know the character of that person (if you are helping yourself, no-one knows yourself better than you do!). It is also important to know the 'character' of the essential oils you think you need (and carrier oils, if used). For emotions which have been living with you for some time, I would suggest 'living with' the oil or oils of your choice for a week at a time, in order to 'experience' your selection and discover which one or ones have the most beneficial effect.

9 *Methods of use*

As I said in Chapter 1, aromatherapy is not just a 'massage using essential oils'; there is *much* more to it than that. If this misinterpretation were truly the case, it would be too time-taking a procedure for problems such as headaches, colds, coughs and numerous other ailments which need instant action.

For essential oils to be effective, they need to be taken into the bloodstream, because once there they can benefit all parts of the body through which the blood itself passes – in other words, everywhere. Essential oils can pass (or be 'carried') into the blood by:

- inhalation; the quickest method, via the brain and lungs, the two main routes (discussed in detail in Chapter 3). This is without doubt the most efficient method of using essential oils to help relieve or release emotions, particularly in cases of panic, shock, anticipated fear (exams, dentist), etc.
- internally; also quick, but needs to be done with care and knowledge, preferably under the direction of an aromatherapist who has had further training specifically in this field (i.e. an aromatologist, *see Useful Addresses*)
- application to the skin; slower than the other two methods, but invaluable where relaxation of the body is of prime importance.

All of these routes need to have a 'vehicle' (called a *carrier*), which will carry the essential oil into the bloodstream. The oils are never, ever used in their concentrated form, except on the skin in emergencies, such as the prevention of a bruise after a knock, a burn, wasp sting, deep cut or burst spot; in these cases only specific oils such as lavender, gully gum eucalyptus (*E. smithii*, **not** *E globulus*), *sweet* marjoram or *sweet* thyme should be used *(see Chapter 8)*. For all other uses (except inhalation, where air is the carrier), essential oils should be mixed into a liquid carrier of some sort, such as water or vegetable oil, as detailed below.

Essential oils are synergistic (from the Greek, *syn* = together and *erg* = work). Each essential oil is a synergistic mix in itself, the chemical components all working together to give the end effect, which is greater than that obtained from the individual components added together (Low, Rawal & Griffin, 1974) – another reason for using only whole, un-tampered-with essential oils. It follows from this that the effect of two or three essential oils added together is also greater than the sum of their individual effects, thus giving you not only increased health benefits – of both mind and body – but also giving you the chance to create an aroma which pleases you.

Synergistic choice of essential oils

Use this chapter to help make a truly synergistic selection of essential oils for, let us say, grief, and bergamot is an aroma you need to use. Out of the 10 properties needed for grief, bergamot possesses six – it is balancing, calming, cicatrizant, digestive, neurotonic and sedative. To make a good synergy, you now need another oil (or oils) to provide the other four. Rosemary, one of the best oils for the emotions, will provide analgesic, cardiotonic, immunostimulant and mentally stimulating properties and frankincense is an effective immunostimulant oil.

Experiment with one drop of each on a tissue, then test the aroma; should it not be exactly to your liking, add another drop of the one that you feel will enhance the aroma for you – or even one drop of another grief oil that you like. The more effort you put into discovering a synergistic mix, the better will be your results!

Making a Blend of Pure Essential Oils

If you decide to use two or more of the same essential oils on a regular basis, it is simpler to mix them together in a small bottle with an integral dropper. From this you can use whatever number of drops you need, in several methods, instead of having to count from separate bottles each time. For instance, should you find that 4 drops of rosemary and 2 each of bergamot and lavender have given you the desired benefits, simply add a nought to the end of each number of drops (40 + 20 + 20 drops) or change the number of drops into ml (4, 2 and 2 ml) if you have a small millilitre measure. Label the bottle!

The following includes all methods and all carriers with which essential oils can be used, as there will no doubt be occasions when you will be experiencing a physical disorder at the same time as you need the essential oils for your emotional problems. Although inhalation (by any method) may give the quickest emotional relief, baths, teas and application (to yourself as well as receiving massage from another person) are also good methods for emotional problems. Remember that *any* method which transports the essential oils into the bloodstream is going to be beneficial!

Air
When you inhale essential oils from a tissue or in a room where they are being vaporized, the concentrated essential oils do not travel up your nose alone – they are in a carrier; the surrounding warm, moist air carries the tiny molecules up the nose as we breathe in. The nose is the only organ with direct access to the brain, which is responsible for influencing our feelings and actions, therefore making the effect of aromas by inhalation exceptionally important.

Tissue
Put 3–6 drops on a tissue for full benefit and, holding this close to your nose, take three really deep breaths. If you or your child have sleeping difficulties, a tissue with essential oils can be put under the pillowcase.

Vaporizer
Put 6–8 drops, with about a tablespoonful of water (depending on the size of the bowl), into the bowl of a vaporizer – I prefer it not to be called a burner, as this suggests an acrid smell; as a matter of fact, if you use a vaporizer without water, you will get an acrid smell when all the lighter molecules of essential oil have evaporated, because the heavy molecules left behind will go sticky and will indeed smell of burning.

Potpourri

Add 8–12 drops of essential oil to some fresh or dried petals in a large screw-top jar. Shake well and leave for an hour or two before shaking again and emptying into a pretty dish or plate. The aroma does not last as long as artificial perfume, but it is much better for your health and it is easy enough to re-shake the petals in the jar with some more essential oil.

Hands

In an emergency, like panic or shock, put one or two drops into the palm of one hand, rub your hands briefly together and cup them over the nose, taking care to keep them away from the eyes. Take one or two deep breaths.

Water

When essential oils are put into warm water, the effects are two-fold because the heat releases the aromatic molecules more quickly. The route the oils take in order to reach the blood circulation depends on the method of use chosen from the following selection.

External Use

Baths

In the bath, molecules of essential oil released into the steam are breathed in, using air as the carrier, and at the same time, the molecules in the water will be carried into the skin of whatever part of the body is in contact with it. Always prepare the bath first, as the extreme heat from the hot tap (which most people run first) would cause the essential oils to evaporate immediately, when they will rise up to the ceiling, leaving very little in the water for you! Use 6–8 drops of essential oil in total (perhaps 3 each of two oils or 3 + 2 + 2 of three oils); they can be added to the bath in various ways, after reaching the required temperature for your comfort:

- drip them directly into the bath, then swish the water well to disperse them thoroughly
- dissolve them first in a little honey or cream, add to the bath and swish well

- make into a thin paste with dried milk, add to the bath and swish well
- put them into a teaspoonful of vegetable oil, add to the bath and swish well; I don't like this method myself, as not only do the bath edges become greasy, but it can eventually make a dirty looking rim if you haven't used detergent on it after every bath.

Foot and Hand Baths
This method is ideal for rheumatic hands and/or feet. Use between 4 and 6 drops in hot water for both foot and hand baths and have a kettle of boiling water beside you to top up as the water starts to cool down. As there are reflex points in both hands and feet, this method could also help other problems, including emotional ones and headaches. Don't forget to swish the water well before putting in your hands or feet to distribute the essential oils evenly.

Sitz Baths
Useful to ease haemorrhoids, stitches after childbirth and for *Candida albicans*. Use 3–4 drops of the appropriate essential oils in your bowl of warm water and sit in the water for 10 minutes; you can keep a kettle of hot water handy in case you need to increase the heat of your water a little.

Compresses
Compresses are successful for a number of problems: insect bites, arthritic joints, period or stomach pains, headaches, sprains, varicose veins, etc. Decide first whether you need a hot or a cold compress; where there is inflammation and heat, a cold compress should be used; for a dull ache, use a warm one. Use a piece of cotton or other natural fibre (handkerchiefs or old cotton or linen tea towels are ideal) just large enough to cover the area to be treated. The size of the container for the water and essential oils should be proportional to the size of the area (for a finger compress an eggcup is big enough). Add your essential oils to just enough water to soak into the compress, adjusting the number of drops according to the size of the area being treated, for example:

- 2 drops for a septic finger
- 8 drops for abdominal pain.

Stir well to disperse the essential oils. Lower the cotton gently into the basin until the water is completely absorbed (squeeze slightly if you have overestimated the amount of water) and lay it onto the problem area, holding in place with a strip of clingfilm. For a warm compress, cover the clingfilm with a scarf or a thermal vest; for a cool one, place a bag of frozen peas (or crushed ice) on the cling film first, changing this when necessary. To keep a compress in place on an arm or leg, a sock or a stocking is ideal. Leave the compress in place for at least an hour or two (overnight for something septic).

Basin of Hot Water
This method is useful for colds, coughs and blocked sinuses. Into a basin of hot water put two or three drops of the relevant essential oils; the reason for so few drops is that the heat of the water accelerates the evaporation of the oils, making the aroma quite strong (so keep your eyes closed), although it will naturally last for a shorter period of time. If you use more drops, especially of peppermint or eucalyptus, the strength of the aroma could make you cough.

Spray
If you don't have a vaporizer, but do have a plant spray bottle, you can spray your room instead. Half-fill the spray bottle with water – warm, if you want a quicker effect – and add 8–12 drops of essential oils. Shake really well before spraying.

Internal Use

When essential oils are to be ingested, it is vital that the oils used are distilled or expressed and are of therapeutic quality (resins and absolutes should not be used). There are so many dubious essential oils on the market that it is difficult to recommend internal use. The decision to use essential oils in this way must therefore be your own, as aromatherapists do not normally prescribe oils for internal use unless they have taken a further qualification in either aromatology or herbal medicine, which gives them the insurance cover to give advice on this use. However, following are two ways you can use *therapeutic quality* (ie unadulterated or organic) essential oils:

Gargles and Mouthwashes

Gargling is an excellent method for a sore throat, or if you think your cold may be going onto your chest. For mouth ulcers, simply swish the oil mixture thoroughly round and round your mouth. Put 2–3 drops of your chosen essential oils into half a glass of water, stir well and take a mouthful. Gargle (or swish) well, before spitting it out. It is important to stir your glass before taking each mouthful as otherwise the essential oils tend to float on the top.

Drinks

Here are a few ideas on making tea and flavouring water with essential oils (for water, shake well, leave for a few hours and shake again each time before use):

- adding 2–3 drops of lemon or orange essential oil to a litre bottle of water gives a pleasant flavour for those people who don't like the bland 'taste' of water
- if you are going to a hot country, take a bottle of fennel with you and put 2–3 drops in your litre of drinking water; it keeps stomach bugs at bay
- if you are seriously making an effort to slim, use 2–3 drops of grapefruit oil (or one of fennel and two of grapefruit) in a litre of water; this must also be accompanied by careful eating.

Bergamot oil is used to flavour commercial Earl Grey tea, so it is easy to make your own (I use tannin-free China tea as the base). To a quarter-pound tin of leaf tea or tea bags scatter 6–8 drops of essential oils and shake the tin well every five or ten minutes for a couple of hours; leave overnight, then make your tea as usual. If the aroma is not strong enough, repeat the shaking process with another 2–3 drops of oil. This tea tastes best (and is better for the health) without the addition of milk.

NB Do not put a drop of essential oil directly into a cup of tea because the taste will be too strong, and the oil will not be effectively dispersed.

I always recommend tea with essential oils to my clients. Not only can you have a variety of flavours, but you can help your own physical and emotional health too by adding the appropriate essential oils:

for example, lemon in the morning to brighten you up and chamomile at night to prepare you for sleep. Also, essential oil bottles take up a lot less room than many different flavours of tea, and in the long run it is less expensive!

This method is helpful for emotional problems, especially ongoing ones. For indigestion and other digestive disorders, like constipation and diarrhoea, a cup of tea two or three times a day is more pleasant than tablets. Urinary tract problems like cystitis react favourably too. I know many people who have found teas to be helpful for the above and also for insomnia and arthritic pain. Remember, however, if you decide to try this method, only use therapeutic quality essential oils – no absolutes or resins.

Application to the Skin

Vegetable oil

The most well-known carriers for this purpose are fixed vegetable oils, into which essential oils readily dissolve. There are many of these on the market, each having its own special benefit to the skin. Do not use mineral oil (beware of some baby oils), as this protects the skin, keeping moisture (urine in the case of baby's nappies) out, therefore it is difficult for essential oils to get in!

Although many people use a vegetable oil for self-application, and sometimes in the bath *(see 'Baths' above)*, the primary purpose of a vegetable carrier oil is for massage; this requires something which allows for continuous and prolonged movement over the body.

To massage the whole body takes between 10–20 ml of vegetable oil, depending on the size (and hairiness!) of the person being massaged. Into this you should put 4–8 drops of your selected essential oils, again depending on the size of the body. It is always better to mix less than you think you will need, rather than more, as the oil left over will contain some of the essential oils which were part of the treatment; however, if all the oil is used, the massage can always be finished with plain carrier oil.

To mix a larger quantity of oil for massage, put 30–40 drops of the chosen essential oils into a 100 ml bottle and add the vegetable oil or oils of your choice to within 2 cm of the top. Screw the lid on firmly and write out a label, with the recipe, the condition it is to help and the date. This makes it easy for you to remake when you need more.

NB When using a vegetable oil mix for self-application, do not pour some into your palm, but place your fingers over the top of the bottle, tipping it up against them. Apply this to the area, repeating the same procedure if you need more oil; this ensures that you will not end up with more oil than you need.

Lotion

When using essential oils on yourself, it is easier to put them into a non-greasy vegetable-based lotion rather than a vegetable oil; this does not stain your clothes as can vegetable oil if you use too much, and it disappears into the skin within a few seconds of applying, leaving your skin soft and smooth, without any greasy feeling.

With an ongoing problem like stress, depression, arthritis or bronchitis, it is preferable to mix a larger quantity (whether the carrier is an oil for massage or a lotion for self-application). For a 100 ml bottle you would need 30–40 drops of the essential oils you have chosen (as for a massage oil). However, the method of mixing is different.

This time, only *some* of the carrier goes into the bottle first, filling only three quarters of the bottle with lotion. Then add the chosen essential oils and shake the bottle well. Finally add the rest of the lotion, up to within 2 cm of the top, to allow you to give the contents a final good shake, to distribute the essential oils evenly.

Cream

You can add essential oils to a cream also, so long as it is a natural, bland, unperfumed base *(see Useful Addresses for products)*. It is easier to relieve symptoms such as chronic sinusitis or persistent headaches at the same time as you moisturize your face and neck, rather than having to apply an extra product as well. For a cream you intend to use every day over a very long period of time, only 3 drops of essential oils in 30 ml of cream are needed.

Storing Essential Oils and Carriers

In perfect storage conditions, essential oils keep far longer than one would think:

- in brown glass bottles
- in a cool place
- without an air space.

If this procedure is followed, essential oils can last about six years, although it is not unknown for them to be in perfect condition after 30–40 years (this is without any air in the bottle). As people would not normally have any oil left after even six years, there is no need to worry about a 'best before' date, so long as the bottling date is known.

Citrus peel oils, because they have not been distilled, have a much shorter life, so it is even more important to regard the storage rules! They can be kept in the fridge, although the waxes (which are not present in distilled oils) may be precipitated. Although this may make the oils appear opaque, it does not affect the therapeutic effect.

When essential oils are mixed into an oil or lotion carrier, the shelf life of that product is limited to the shelf life of the carrier used, and the storage rules regarding light, heat and firm closure are even more relevant:

- in a vegetable carrier oil, keeping qualities are reduced to around 12 months as the vegetable oil will eventually go rancid; this is not believed to hinder the effects of the essential oil, but the aroma takes on a rancid note
- in a natural lotion *(see Useful Addresses)* the keeping qualities are the same as that of the pure essential oil on its own – at least 6 years – when kept in the correct conditions.

Caution: Never leave a bottle of pure essential oil on a polished or enamelled surface (or certain types of plastic such as that used for cassettes) as these may react with the chemicals in the oil and be damaged.

Conclusion

All the methods given in this chapter are relatively simple, involving only a little effort by the individual concerned. Active participation plays an important part in one's own cure (in any sort of disease), particularly where the problems are emotional, as the power of the mind is focussed on the healing aspect; thus the whole healing process is accelerated.

I must emphasize that the ingestion of essential oils as medicines is only to be carried out under the direction of a practitioner qualified in this field.

Epilogue

You will have read through this book and responded to it emotionally – there is no-one in life who is not susceptible to feelings; all of us are different and none of us is unchangeable. You may not always agree with some of my thoughts, theories and ideas and you will no doubt think of other essential oil properties which may help each emotion I have illustrated (as I have myself on reading through, though these will have to wait for a second edition!). Nevertheless, I trust you have enjoyed reading it as much as I have enjoyed writing it.

References

Chapter 1

'Human emotion: emotions and adaptation'. 1996 *Encyclopaedia Britannica*, Inc. CD ROM

Borysenko, J. 1988 *Minding the Body, Mending the Mind*. Bantam, Toronto: 176–7

Bradburn, N.M. 1969 *The Structure of Psychological Well-being*. Aldean, Chicago

Gerber, R. 1988 *Vibrational Medicine*. Bear & Co., Sante Fé, CA: 470

Grounds, V.C. 1999 *Whose Business? Our Daily Bread*. RBC Ministries, Michigan, Vol. 44, 4: July 5th

Hay, L.L. 1988 *You Can Heal Your Life*. Eden Grove Editions, London

Knasko, S. 1997 'Ambient odour'. *International Journal of Aromatherapy*, Vol. 8, no 3: 28–33

Lindenfield, G. 1998 *Emotional Confidence*. Thorsons, London

McLeod, W.T. (chief editor) 1981 *Pocket Dictionary of the English Language*. Collins, London

Merriam-Webster 1994 *Merriam-Webster's Collegiate Dictionary*. CD ROM

Price, S. 1991 *Aromatherapy for Common Ailments*. Gaia, London: 16

Price, S. 1993 *The Aromatherapy Workbook*. Thorsons, London: 178

Rochfort, J. 1998 'Counselling therapy – an emotional approach'. *Aromatherapy Times* 5–6

Schwartz, C. (chief editor) 1991 *Chambers Concise Dictionary*. Chambers, Edinburgh

Stephen, R. 1999 personal communication

Stephen, R. 1998 'Aromatherapy and bereavement'. *The Aromatherapist*, Vol. 5, no.2: 8–16

Vander Lugt 1999. 'How accountable are you?' *Our Daily Bread*. RBC Ministries, Michigan, Vol. 44, 4: July 16th

Vernon, H. 1998 personal communication

Vieth, I. (ed.) 199? *The Yellow Emperor's Classic of Internal Medicine*. Pelanduk, Malaysia

Wingate, P. and Wingate, R. 1988 *The Penguin Medical Encyclopedia*. Penguin Books, London

Wood, C. 1990 *Say Yes to Life*. Dent, London

Chapter 2

Baron, R.A. 1990 'Environmentally induced positive affect: its impact on self efficacy, task performance, negotiation and conflict'. *Journal of Applied Social Psychology* 16: 16–28

Bennett, G.E. 1989 'The body/mind relationship'. *Health consciousness*, Vol. X, no 4: 27–31

Ehrlichman, H. and Bastone, L. 1992 'The use of odour in the study of emotion'. *Fragrance: The Psychology and Biology of Perfume*: 143–59

Hartvig, K. and Rowley, N. 1996 *You Are What You Eat*. Piatkus, London

Hay. L.L. 1988 *You Can Heal Your Life*. Eden Grove Editions, London

Hooper, A. 1988 *Massage and Loving*. Unwin Hyman, London

Montague, A. 1986 *Touching – The Human Significance of the Skin*. Harper and Row, New York

Nash, J.M. 1997 'Fertile minds'. *Time*, February 10th: 48–58

Price, S. 1993 *Aromatherapy Workbook*. Thorsons, London: 177

Wallace, P.A. 1999 'The raphae formula development'. *Nature's Own News* (supplement), September issue

Warren, C. and Warrenburg, S. 1993 'Mood benefits of fragrance'. *International Journal of Aromatherapy*, Vol. 5, no. 2: 12–16

Chapter 3

Badia, P., Westensen, N., Lammers, W., Culpepper, J. and Harsh, J. 1990 'Responsiveness of olfactory stimuli presented in sleep'. *Psychology and Behaviour* 48, 1:87–90

Buchbauer, G. 1993 'Molecular interaction'. *The International Journal of Aromatherapy*, 5,3: 11–14

Classen, C., Howes, D. and Synott, A. 1994 *Aroma: the Cultural History of Smell*. Routledge, London: 2

Dodd, G.H. and Skinner, M. 1992 'From moods to molecules: the psychopharmacology of perfumery and aromatherapy'. In van Toller, S. and Dodd, G.H. *Fragrance: The Psychology and Biology of Perfume*. Elsevier, London

Fischer-Rizzi, S. 1990 *The Complete Aromatherapy Handbook*. Sterling, New York: 27

Gatti, G. and Cayola, R. 1923 'Azione terapeutica degli olii essenziali'. *Rivista Italiana delle Essenze e Profumi* 5 (12): 133–5

Genders, R. 1972 *A History of Scent*. Hamish Hamilton, London: 3

Holley, A. 1993 'Actualité du méchamismede l'olfaction'. *12èmes Journées Internationales Huiles Essentielles*. Istituo Tethahedron, Milan: 21–7

Kirk-Smith, M.D., van Toller, S. and Dodd, G.H. 1983 'Unconscious odour conditioning in human subjects'. *Biological Psychology* 17:221–32

Lawless, J. 1994 *Aromatherapy and the Mind*. Thorsons, London: 14

Lawson, 1995 personal communication

Nasel, B., Nasel, C., Samec, P., Schindler, E. and Buchbauer, G. 1994 'Functional imaging of effects of fragrances on the human brain after prolonged inhalation'. *Chemical Senses* 19,4:359–64

Ohloff, G. 1944 *Scent and Fragrances*. Springer-Verlag, Berlin: IX

Price, L. and S. 1999 *Aromatherapy for Health Professionals*. Churchill Livingstone, Edinburgh

Price, S. 1991 *Aromatherapy for Common Ailments*. Gaia, London: 16

Rowe, V.L. 1999 personal communication

Sacks, O. 1987 *The Man who Mistook his Wife for a Hat*. Duckworth, London: 159

Schmidt, H-O 1995 'Fragrance & health: observations on aromachology'. *H&R Contact* 61: 16–20

Süskind, P. 1986 *Perfume: the story of a murderer*. Hamish Hamilton, London

Torii, S., Fukuda, H., Kanemoto, H., Miyauchi, R., Hamauzu, Y. and Kawasaki, M. 1988 'Contingent negative variation and the psychological effects of odour'. In *Perfumery: The Psychology and Biology of Fragrance*. Chapman & Hall, London: 107–20

Turin, L. 1995 'A code in the nose'. Text adapted from *Horizon* programme, transmitted 27 November. BBC, London van Toller, S. 1993 'The sensory evaluation of odours'. Lecture notes, Clinical Practitioner's Course. Shirley Price International College of Aromatherapy: 3

Warren, C. and Warrenburg, S. 1993 'Mood benefits of fragrance'. *International Journal of Aromatherapy* 5,2:12–16

Williams, D. 1996 *The Chemistry of Essential Oils*. Micelle, Weymouth: 27

Wysocki, C.J., Beauchamp, G.K., Todrank, J. and Pierce, J.D. 1992 'Individual sufferances in olfactory ability'. In van Toller, S. and Dodd, G.H. *Fragrance: The Psychology and Biology of Perfume*. Elsevier, London: 99–101

Chapter 4

Bennett, G. 1989 'The body/mind relationship'. *Health Consciousness*, Vol. X, no. 4: 27–31

Borysenko, J. 1988 *Minding the Body, Mending the Mind*. Bantam, Toronto: 12–13

Chen, N.K. 1986 'The epidemiology of self-perceived fatigue among adults'. *Preventive Medicine* 15: 74–81

Cousins, N. 1979 *Anatomy of an Illness as Perceived by a Patient*. Norton, New York

Editorial 1884 *British Medical Journal*: 1: 1163

Everett, A. 1973 'Mind dynamics'. Course notes.

Gerber, G. 1988 *Vibrational Medicine*. Bear & Co, Santa Fé CA: 379–80

Infante, A. 1986 *Sing your way to health, wealth and happiness*. Relaxation Centre, Car Brooke and Wickham Sts. Fortitude Valley, Queensland 4006, Australia

Maltby, J., Lewis, C.A. and Day, L. 1999 'Religious orientation and psychological well-being: the role of the frequency of personal prayer'. *The British Journal of Health Psychology*, Vol. 4 (4): 363–78

Peale, N.V. 1992 *The Power of Positive Thinking*. Cedar, London: 1

Price, L. and Price, S. 1999 *Aromatherapy for Health Professionals*. Churchill Livingstone, Edinburgh: 158

Steele, J. 1984 'Brain research and essential oils'. *Aromatherapy Quarterly*: Spring issue

Torii, S. *et al* 1988 'Contingent negative variation and the psychological effects of odour'. In *Perfumery: The Psychology and Biology of Fragrance*. Chapman and Hall, London: 107–20

Wingate, P. and Wingate, R. *The Penguin Medical Encyclopaedia.* Penguin Books, London: 336

Wood, C. 1990 *Say Yes to Life.* Dent, London

Chapter 5

Boyd, E.M. and Pearson, G.L. 1946 'The expectorant action of volatile oils'. *American Journal of Medical Science* 211:602–10

Buchbauer, G., Jirovetz, L., Jäger, W., Plank, C. and Dietrich, H. 1993 'Fragrance compounds and essential oils with sedative effects upon inhalation'. *Journal of Pharmaceutical Sciences* 82 (6) (June): 660–64

Debelmas, A.M. and Rochat, J. 1964 'Etude comparée sur la fibre lisse des solutions aqueuse saturées d'essence de thym, de thymol et de carvacrol'. *Bulletin des Travaux.* Société de Pharmacies de Lyon 4: 163–72

Debelmas, A.M. and Rochat, J. 1967 'Activité antispasmodique étudiée sur une cinquante d'echantillons differents'. *Plantes Médicinales et Phytothérapie* 1: 23–7

Franchomme, P. and Pénoël, D. 1990 *L'aromathérapie exactement.* Jallois, Limoges: 283–4

Gordonoff, T. 1938 'Ergebnisse der Physiologie, biologischen Chemie und experimentallen'. *Pharmakologie* 40:53

Jakovlev, V., Isaac, O. and Flascamp, E. 1983 'Pharmacological investigations with compounds of chamomile. VI. Investigations on the antiphlogistic effects of chamazulene and matricin'. *Planta Medica* 49: 67–73

Larrondo, J.V. and Calvo, M.A. 1991 'Effect of essential oils on *Candida albicans:* a scanning electron microscope study'. *Biomed letters* 46, 184:269–72

Maruzella, J.C. 1961 'Antifungal properties of perfume oils'. *Journal of the American Pharmaceutical Association* 50:655

Price, S. 1999 *Practical Aromatherapy* (4th edition). Thorsons, London: 57

Price, L. and Price, S. 1999 *Aromatherapy for Health Professionals.* Churchill Livingstone, Edinburgh

Rossi, T., Melegari, M., Bianchi, A., Albasini, A. and Vampa, G. 1988 'Sedative, antiinflammatory and antidiuretic effects induced in rats by essential oil of vanities of *Anthemis nobilis*: a comparative study'.

Pharmacology Research Communications 5 (December 20): 71–4

Schilcher, H. 1985 'Effects and side effects of essential oils'. In Baerheim Svendsen, A. and Scheffer, J.J.C. (eds) *Essential Oils and Aromatic Plants*. Martinus Nijhof/Junk, Dordrecht

Taddei, I., Giachetti, D., Taddei, E., Mantovani, P. and Bianchi, E. 1988 'Spasmolytic activity of peppermint, sage and rosemary essences and their major constituents'. *Fitoterapia* 59: 463–8

Thompson, D.P. and Cannon, C. 1986 'Toxicity of essential oils on toxigenic and nontoxigenic fungi'. *Bulletin of Environmental Contamination and Toxicology* 36, 4, April: 527–32

Torii, S. *et al* 1988 'Contingent negative variation and the psychological effects of odour'. In *Perfumery: The psychology and biology of fragrance*. Chapman and Hall, London: 107–20

Weiss, R.F. 1988 *Herbal Medicine*. Arcanum, Göteborg: 296

Woolfson, A. and Hewitt, D. 1992 'Intensive aromacare'. *International Journal of Aromatherapy* 4 (2): 12–13

Chapter 6

Brown, G.W. and Harris, T. 1978 *Social Origins of Depression*. Tavistock, London

Carter, R. 1998 *Mapping the Mind*. Weidenfeld & Nicholson, London: 99–100

Domar, A.D. and Dreher, H. 1997 *Healing Mind, Healthy Woman*. Thorsons, London: 159

Lindenfield, G. 1997 *Emotional Confidence*. Thorsons, London: 21

Martin, M. and Clark, D.M. 1985 'Cognitive mediation of depressed mood and neuroticism'. *IRCS Medical Science* 13: 352–3

Price, L. 1994 'Stress and depression – the major causes of hair loss'. Unpublished paper.

Price, L. and Price, S. 1999 *Aromatherapy for Health Professionals*. Churchill Livingstone, Edinburgh: 208

Selye, H. 1984 *The Stress of Life*. McGraw Hill, New York: xvi & 1

Topping, W.W. 1990 *Success over Distress*. Topping International Institute, Bellingham, WA: 1

Warren, C. and Warrenburg, S. 1993 'Mood benefits of fragrance'. *International Journal of Aromatherapy* 5,2:12–16

Wingate P. and Wingate R. *The Penguin Medical Encyclopedia*. Penguin Books, London: 453

Wood, C. 1990 *Say Yes to Life*. Dent, London
Yoder, J.E. 1999 'Love by listening'. *Our Daily Bread*, RBC Ministries, Carnforth, Lancs: October 1st

Chapter 7

Battaglia, S. 1997 *The Complete Guide to Aromatherapy*. The Perfect Potion, Australia
Birmingham Post. 'Shame on us'. Cited in *Reader's Digest* 1997 December: 116
Chance, A. 'Fear'. *Aromatherapy Quarterly* 57: 39
Culpeper, N. (Date not given) *Culpeper's Complete Herbal*. Foulsham, Slough: 36–37
Davis, P. 1991 *Subtle Aromatherapy*. Daniel, Saffron Walden: 209
Domar, A.D. and Dreher, H. 1997 *Healing Mind, Healthy Woman*. Thorsons, London
Eccles, S. 1995 Editorial. *Aromatherapy Quarterly* 45: 2
Fewkes, M. 1998 'Journal jottings'. *The Aromatherapist*, Vol. 5, no 1: 34–7
Fischer-Rizzi, S. 1990 *The Complete Aromatherapy Handbook*. Sterling, New York
Hay, L.L. 1988 *You Can Heal Your Life*. Eden Grove Editions, London: 159
Holmes, P. 1992 'Lavender oil'. *International Journal of Aromatherapy*, Vol. 4 (2): 20–22
Keville, K. and Green, M. 1995 *Aromatherapy. A Complete Guide to the Healing Art*. The Crossing Press, Freedom, CA
Lawless, J. 1994 *Aromatherapy and the Mind*. Thorsons, London
Lindenfield, G. 1997 *Emotional Confidence*. Thorsons, London
McCasland, D.C. 1999 'Hostile heart'. *Our Daily Bread*. RBC Ministries, Michigan: Vol. 44: September 7th
Mojay, G. 1996 *Aromatherapy for Healing the Spirit*. Gaia Books, London
Murray-Parkes, C. 1986 *Bereavement: Studies of Grief in Adult Life*. Pelican, London
Price, L. and Price, S. 1999 *Aromatherapy for Health Professionals*. Churchill Livingstone, Edinburgh
Robinson, J.C.T. 1948 'The fear problem – some ways of regarding it'. Lecture to the British Psychological Society, unpublished paper

Scnaubelt, K. 1998 *Medical Aromatherapy*. Frog Ltd, Berkeley, CA: 94
Stephen, R. 1998 'Aromatherapy and bereavement'. *The Aromatherapist*, Vol. 5, no.2: 8–16
Veith, I. (ed.) 1992 *The Yellow Emperor's Classic of Internal Medicine*. Pelanduk, Malaysia: 42, 107
Wingate, P. and Wingate, R. *The Penguin Medical Encyclopedia*. Penguin Books, London
Wood, C. 1990 *Say Yes to Life*. Dent, London: 49
Zevon, M.A. and Tellegen, A. 1982 'The structure of mood change: an idiographic/nomothetic analysis'. *Journal of Personality and Social Psychology* 43: 111–22

Chapter 8
Bourret, J.C. 1981 *Les Nouveaux Sices de la Medicine par les Plantes*. Hachette, Paris: 281
Burrough, R. 1999 Lecture report. *Herbs*, Vol. 24, no. 3: 22
Clair, C. 1961 *Of Herbs and Spices*. Abelard–Schuman, London: 219
Collin, P. 1997 'Niaouli' (translated by Len Price). *The Aromatherapist*, Vol. 4, No. 2
Davis, P. *Aromatherapy: an A-Z*. Daniel, London: 191–2
Fischer-Rizzi, S. 1990 *The Complete Aromatherapy Handbook*. Sterling, New York
Gerard, J. 1964 *Gerard's Herbal*. Spring Books, London: 156
Grieve, M. 1998 *A Modern Herbal*. Tiger Books, Twickenham
Law, D. 1982 *The Concise Herbal Encyclopedia*. Bartholomew, Edinburgh: 63
Lawless, J. 1994 *Aromatherapy and the Mind*. Thorsons, London
Mabey, R. *The Complete New Herbal*. Elm Tree Books, London: 69
Maury, M. 1989 *Marguerite Maury's Guide to Aromatherapy*. Daniel, Saffron Walden: 87
Price, S. and Price Parr, P. 1996 *Aromatherapy for Babies and Children*. Thorsons, London: 26
Price, S. 1991 *Aromatherapy for common ailments*. Gaia, London: 8
Price. L. Price, S. and Smith, I. 2000 *Carrier Oils for Aromatherapy and Massage*. Riverhead, Stratford-upon-Avon
Schnaubelt, K. 1993 'Aromatherapy and chronic viral infections'. (Conference proceedings, *Aroma* 1993) Aromatherapy Publications, Hove: 37

Valnet, J. 1980 *The Practice of Aromatherapy*. Daniel, Saffron Walden: 120

Chapter 9
Low, D., Rawal, B.D. and Griffin, W.J. 1974 'Antibacterial action of the essential oils of some Australian Myrtaceae with special references to the activity of chromatographic fractions of oil of *Eucalyptus citriodora*'. *Planta Medica* 26: 184–9

Useful Addresses

Aromatherapy products

Great Britain
Shirley Price Aromatherapy Ltd
Essentia House
Upper Bond Street
Hinckley
Leics LE10 1RS
Tel: 01455 615466
Fax: 01455 615054

Herbal Garden
20 Eldon Gardens
Percy Street
Newcastle
Tyne & Wear

Herbal Garden
93 Rose Street
Edinburgh
Lothian EH2 3DT

Training

Aromatherapy
Shirley Price International College
 of Aromatherapy Ltd
Address as above
Tel: 01455 633231

The S.E.E.D. Institute
Therapeutic Division
10 Magnolia Way
Fleet
Hants GU13 9JZ

Aromatherapy and specialized short courses
Penny Price
Sketchley Manor
Burbage
Leics LE10 2LQ
Fax: 01455 617972

Aromatic medicine and aromatology
Robert Stephen (consultant)
4 Woodland Road
Hinckley
Leics LE10 1JG
Tel/Fax: 01455 611829

Aromatic medicine association
The Institute of Aromatic Medicine
 (IAM)
Aromed House
41 Leicester Road
Hinckley
Leics LE10 1LW

Aromatherapy Associations

Aromatherapy Organisations Council (AOC)
PO Box 19834
London SE25 6WF
Tel: 020 8251 7912
Fax: 020 8251 7942

International Society of Professional Aromatherapists (ISPA)
ISPA House
82 Ashby Road
Hinckley
Leics LE10 1SN
Tel: 01455 647987
Fax: 01455 890956

International Federation of Aromatherapists (IFA)
Stamford House
2/4 Chiswick High Road
London W4 1TH
Tel: 020 8742 2605
Fax: 020 8742 2606

Aromatherapy training and products

Australia
Australian School of Awareness
PO Box 187
Montrose
Victoria 3765
Australia
Tel: (03) 9723 2509
Fax: (03) 9761 8895

Israel
Fern Allen
PO Box 4363
Jerusalem
Israel
Tel: 00 972 267 9908

Italy
Jenny Bird
Via Vigevano 43
Milan 20144
Italy
Tel: 00 39 258 113261

Northern Ireland
European College of Natural Therapies
16 North Parade
Belfast BT7 2GG
Northern Ireland
Tel: 028 9064 1454

Republic of Ireland
Mary Cavanagh
Chamomile
Three Mile Water
Wicklow
Eire
Tel: 00 353 404 47219
Fax: 00 353 404 47319

Christine Courtney
Oban Aromatherapy
53 Beech Grove
Lucan
Co. Dublin
Eire
Tel: 00 353 1628 2121

Norway
Margareth Thomte
Nedreslottsgate 25
0157 Oslo
Norway
Tel: 00 47 22 170017
Fax: 00 47 22 425777

Switzerland
Sara Gelzer
Eigentalstr 552 No 14
8425 Oberembrach
Switzerland
Tel: 00 41 1 865 4996

USA

Training and products

Nordblom Swedish Healthcare Centre
178 Mill Creek Road
Livingstone
Montana 59047
USA
Tel: 001 406 333 4216
Fax: 001 406 333 4415

Training

The Australasian College of Herbal
  Studies
PO Box 57
Lake Oswego
Oregon 97034
USA
Tel: 001 503 635 6652
Fax: 001 503 697 0615

R J Buckle Associates
PO Box 868
Hunter
NY 12442
USA
Tel: 001 518 263 4405
Fax: 001 518 263 4031

Aromatherapy Association

National Association for Holistic
  Aromatherapy
PO Box 17622
Boulder
Colorado 80308 – 7622
USA
Tel: 001 888-ASK-NAHA
Tel: 001 314 963 2071
Fax: 001 314 963 4454

Stockists only

Northern Ireland
Angela Hillis
32 Russell Park
Belfast
Co. Antrim BT5 7QW
Northern Ireland

Iceland
Bergfell ehf
Skipholt 50c
105 Reykjavik
Iceland
Tel: 00 354 551 5060
Fax: 00 354 551 5065

Japan
Oz International Ltd
K5 Building
6F 4–5 Kojimachi
Chiyodaleu
Tokyo 102–0083
Japan
Tel: 00 81 3 5213 3060
Fax: 00 81 3 3262 1970

Korea
Jung Dong Cosmetics Co Ltd
501 Shinham Officetel
49–5 Chungdam-Dong
Kangnam-Ku
Seoul
Korea

Malta
Professional Health & Beauty Services
Comflor APT
1B Marfa Road
Mellieha Bay
SPB10 Malta

Singapore
Eden Marketing Pte
63 Hillview Avenue
09–21 Lam Soon Industrial Building
Singapore 2366
Tel: 00 65 7696168
Fax: 00 65 7693937

Taiwan
Chun Hun
8F, No 205, Sec. 1
Fu-Shin S. Road
Taipei
Taiwan
Tel: 00 886 2751 3590
Fax: 00 886 2776 3547/1599

Jong Yeong Cosmetics Co Ltd
16 Tze Chyang 3rd Road
Nan Kang Industry Park
Nan Tou
Taiwan
Tel: 00 886 49 251065
Fax: 00 886 49 251071

Index